Study Guide for Understanding Nursing Research
Building an Evidence-Based Practice

Seventh Edition

Susan K. Grove and Jennifer R. Gray

Study Guide prepared by

Susan K. Grove, PhD, RN, ANP-BC, GNP-BC

Professor Emerita
College of Nursing and Health Innovation
The University of Texas at Arlington
Arlington, Texas;
Adult Nurse Practitioner Consultant

Jennifer R. Gray, PhD, RN, FAAN

Associate Dean, College of Natural and Health Sciences
Oklahoma Christian University
Oklahoma City, Oklahoma;
Professor Emerita
College of Nursing and Health Innovation
The University of Texas at Arlington
Arlington, Texas

Christy Bomer-Norton, PhD, RN, CNM, IBCLC

Consultant
Concord, Massachusetts

ELSEVIER

ELSEVIER

3251 Riverport Lane
St. Louis, Missouri 63043

Study Guide for Understanding Nursing Research
Building an Evidence-Based Practice, SEVENTH EDITION

ISBN: 978-0-323-53204-4

Notices

Practitioners and researchers must always rely on their own experience and knowledge in evaluating and using any information, methods, compounds or experiments described herein. Because of rapid advances in the medical sciences, in particular, independent verification of diagnoses and drug dosages should be made. To the fullest extent of the law, no responsibility is assumed by Elsevier, authors, editors or contributors for any injury and/or damage to persons or property as a matter of products liability, negligence or otherwise, or from any use or operation of any methods, products, instructions, or ideas contained in the material herein.

Content Strategist: Lee Henderson
Content Development Manager: Lisa Newton
Content Development Specialist: Laurel Shea
Publishing Services Manager: Shereen Jameel
Project Manager: Radhika Sivalingam
Cover Designer: Muthukumaran Thangaraj

Printed in the United States of America
Last digit is the print number: 9 8 7 6 5 4 3 2

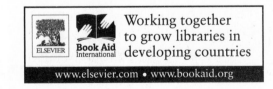

Working together
to grow libraries in
developing countries

www.elsevier.com • www.bookaid.org

To the nursing students who are our next generation of researchers essential for building an evidence-based practice for nursing.

Susan, Jennifer, and Christy

In loving memory of my sister Sheryl A. Grove, my best friend, supporter, and mentor.

Susan

To my husband, Randy, for supporting my scholarly goals.

Jennifer

To my husband, Matthew, for your unwavering love and support.

Christy

We hope that this Study Guide is helpful to you in learning the steps of the research process, critically appraising studies, and synthesizing research findings to facilitate an evidence-based practice for your patients and their families.

Susan K. Grove,
Jennifer R. Gray
Christy Bomer-Norton

Reviewers

Karen E. Alexander, PhD, RN, CNOR
Program Director RN-BSN, Assistant Professor
Department of Nursing
University of Houston-Clear Lake
Pearland
Houston, Texas

Sara L. Clutter, PhD, RN
Professor of Nursing
Department of Nursing
Waynesburg University
Waynesburg, Pennsylvania

Deborah A. Lekan, PhD, RN-BC
Assistant Professor
Department of Family and Community Health Nursing
University of North Carolina at Greensboro School of
  Nursing
Greensboro, North Carolina

Preface

The knowledge generated through nursing research is rapidly expanding each year. This empirical knowledge is critical for developing an evidence-based practice in nursing that is both high quality and cost-effective for patients, families, providers, and healthcare agencies. As a nursing student and registered nurse, you will be encouraged to read, critically appraise, and use research findings to develop protocols, algorithms, and policies for practice. We recognize that learning research terminology and reading and critically appraising research reports are complex and sometimes overwhelming activities. Thus we have developed this *Study Guide for Understanding Nursing Research* to assist you in clarifying, comprehending, analyzing, synthesizing, and applying the content presented in your textbook, *Understanding Nursing Research*, 7th edition.

The Study Guide is organized into 14 chapters, which are consistent with the chapters of the textbook. Each chapter presents you with learning exercises that require various levels of knowledge and critical thinking skills. These exercises are organized using the following headings: Terms and Definitions, Linking Ideas, Web-Based Information and Resources, and Conducting Critical Appraisals to Build an Evidence-Based Practice. In some exercises, you will define relevant terms or identify key ideas. In other exercises, you will demonstrate comprehension of the research process by linking one idea to another. Another section was developed with exercises to increase your use of web-based resources to locate relevant research information for classroom and clinical activities. In the most complex exercises, you will apply your new research knowledge by conducting critical appraisals of published quantitative and qualitative studies.

This edition of the Study Guide has been updated, refined, and condensed to include essential research knowledge for baccalaureate nursing students and registered nurses. Current, relevant content has been provided for understanding the following steps of the quantitative research process: problem, purpose, literature review, framework, ethics, design, sampling, measurement, statistics, and findings. We have updated the content on the following four types of qualitative research commonly conducted in nursing: phenomenology, grounded theory research, ethnographic research, and exploratory-descriptive qualitative research. The textbook also includes revised and simplified critical appraisal processes for quantitative and qualitative research, and these processes are applied to a current qualitative study and a quantitative study throughout this Study Guide. You also are provided exercises to facilitate your reading of syntheses of research and using this knowledge in developing evidence-based protocols, algorithms, and policies in clinical agencies. New to the 7th edition of the textbook and study guide is a focus on understanding mixed methods research. This study guide includes a mixed methods study that is critically appraised in selected chapters, with a comprehensive appraisal of the study provided in Chapter 14.

After completing the exercises for each chapter, you will be able to review the answers in the Answer Key at the back of the book to assess your understanding of the content. Based on your correct and incorrect responses, you will be able to focus your study to improve your knowledge of each chapter's content. We believe that completing the exercises in the Study Guide will improve your performance in the classroom and during clinical experiences. We also think this Study Guide can provide you with a background for reading, analyzing, and synthesizing the evidence from research reports for application to practice.

HOW TO GET THE MOST OUT OF THIS STUDY GUIDE

The exercises in *Study Guide for Understanding Nursing Research*, 7th edition, are designed to assist you in comprehending the content in your textbook, conducting critical appraisals of nursing studies, and using research knowledge to promote an evidence-based practice. Thus you will need to read each chapter in your text before completing the chapters in this Study Guide. Begin by scanning the entire chapter to get an overall view of the content. Then read the textbook chapter with the intent of increasing your comprehension of each section. As you examine each section, pay careful attention to the terms that are defined. If the meaning of a term is not clear to you, look up its definition in the Glossary and identify other pages on which the term is used in the Index at the back of the textbook. Highlight key ideas in each section. Examine tables and figures as they are referenced in the text. Mark sections that you do not sufficiently understand. Jot down questions to ask your instructor in class or to post to your course discussion board.

After carefully reading a chapter in the text, complete the Study Guide exercises; this will assist you in learning relevant content. Each Study Guide chapter includes four major headings, which are discussed as follows.

Exercise 1: Terms and Definitions

This section of each Study Guide chapter consists of a matching test of key terms and their definitions. Key terms are identified in color in the text and defined within the chapters to assist you in becoming familiar with essential terminology for understanding the research process. As you read the text, do not skip over terms in the chapter that are unfamiliar to you. Instead, mark unfamiliar words as you read and look up their definitions in the Glossary at the end of the text. Being familiar with the terms will increase your ability to comprehend the course content, contribute to class or online discussions, apply your new knowledge, and critically appraise studies.

Exercise 2: Linking Ideas

This section of each Study Guide chapter helps you identify important information and link relevant ideas in each textbook chapter. Completing the fill-in-the-blank and matching questions will prompt you to review and analyze the content of the chapter, which is the key to comprehending and applying content related to the research process in educational and clinical activities. You may need to refer to specific sections, tables, and figures in the text to complete some of these questions.

Exercise 3: Web-Based Information and Resources

Each chapter in the Study Guide includes questions that require you to access online materials for answers. These questions are provided to introduce you to the wealth of information that is available online related to research and evidence-based practice. Many of these resources are valuable websites that you may want to bookmark for use in other courses and following graduation.

Exercise 4: Conducting Critical Appraisals to Build an Evidence-Based Practice

Critical appraisal exercises are provided to give you experiences in appraising published nursing studies. In some cases, brief quotes are provided, with questions addressing information specific to the chapter content. The majority of the critical appraisal exercises focus on the three published studies that are provided in Appendices A, B, and C of this Study Guide. One study is quantitative, another is qualitative, and the third is mixed methods (see Published Studies section). By completing the Study Guide, you can incorporate the critical appraisal information you have learned to perform an overall critical appraisal of these three studies. In addition, you can take the knowledge you have gained and apply it in the critical appraisal of other published quantitative, qualitative, and mixed methods studies.

Answer Key

The answers to all Study Guide questions are provided in the Answer Key in the back of the Study Guide. We recommend that you not refer to these answers except to check your own responses to the questions. You will learn more by reading the textbook and searching for the answers on your own.

Published Studies

Reprints of three published studies are provided in Appendices A, B, and C. The Hallas, Koslap-Petraco, and Fletcher (2017) study is an experimental quantitative study with the design of a randomized controlled trial. The Erikson and Davies (2017) study is a grounded theory qualitative study; and the Wendler, Smith, Ellenburg, Gill, Anderson, and Spiegel-Thayer (2017) study is a mixed methods study. These studies are referenced in many of the questions throughout the Study Guide. Additional published studies referenced in the Study Guide are found in the Research Article Library of the online resources for this textbook at https://evolve.elsevier.com/grove/understanding/.

   Additional online questions and exercises (available at https://evolve.elsevier.com/grove/understanding/) have been developed to further enhance your understanding of the research process. You are now ready to begin your adventure of learning about the research process to build an evidence-based practice.

Contents

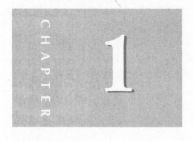

Introduction to Nursing Research and Its Importance in Building an Evidence-Based Practice

INTRODUCTION

You need to read Chapter 1 and then complete the following exercises. These exercises will assist you in learning key research terms, understanding the historical development of research in nursing, describing how knowledge is acquired in nursing, identifying the research methods conducted in nursing, understanding your role in nursing research, and determining the best research evidence for practice. The answers to these exercises are in the Answer Key at the back of the book.

EXERCISE 1: TERMS AND DEFINITIONS

Acquiring Knowledge and Research Methods

Directions: Match each term below with its correct definition. Each term is used only once and all terms are defined.

Terms

a. Borrowing
b. Deductive reasoning
c. Explanation
d. Inductive reasoning
e. Intuition
f. Knowledge
g. Mixed methods research
h. Nursing research

i. Outcomes research
j. Personal experience
k. Prediction
l. Qualitative research
m. Quality and Safety Education for Nurses (QSEN)
n. Quantitative research
o. Role modeling
p. Trial and error

Definitions

_____ 1. Essential information acquired in a variety of ways that is expected to be an accurate reflection of reality and is used to direct a person's actions.

_____ 2. A scientific process that validates and refines existing knowledge and generates new knowledge that directly and indirectly influences nursing practice.

_____ 3. Reasoning from the specific to the general, such as reasoning from a specific symptom to the nursing diagnosis of acute pain.

_____ 4. Gaining knowledge by being actively involved in a situation, such as providing care to elderly patients in an intensive care unit (ICU).

_____ 5. A formal, objective, systematic research process to describe, test relationships, or examine cause-and-effect interactions among variables.

_____   6. Reasoning from the general to the specific or from a general premise to a particular situation.

_____   7. An approach with unknown outcomes that is used in a situation of uncertainty when other sources of knowledge are unavailable.

_____   8. Insight or understanding of a situation or event as a whole that usually cannot be logically explained, such as knowing that a patient's life is in jeopardy.

_____   9. A systematic, interactive, subjective research approach used to describe life experiences and give them meaning.

_____   10. Knowledge generated from research that clarifies relationships among variables.

_____   11. An important scientific methodology that was developed to examine the results of patient care, such as length of hospital stay, morbidity rate, mortality rate, and quality of life.

_____   12. Knowledge generated from research that enables one to estimate the probability of a specific outcome in a given situation, such as the probability of an elderly patient falling during hospitalization.

_____   13. An approach to inquiry that combines quantitative and qualitative research methods in a single study.

_____   14. Learning by imitating the behaviors of an expert, such as the process of faculty teaching students by demonstrating appropriate behaviors.

_____   15. The appropriation and use of knowledge from other disciplines like medicine and psychology to guide nursing practice.

_____   16. A professional nursing initiative that identified the requisite knowledge, skills, and attitudes (KSAs) for the competencies of pre-licensure education.

Evidence-Based Practice Terms

Directions: Match each term below with its correct definition. Each term is used only once and all terms are defined.

Terms
a. Best research evidence
b. Clinical expertise
c. Critical appraisal of research
d. Evidence-based guidelines
e. Evidence-based practice (EBP)

Definitions

_____   1. The integration of best research evidence with our clinical expertise and patients' circumstances and values to produce quality health outcomes.

_____   2. Knowledge and skills of the healthcare professional providing care; determined for a nurse by years of clinical experience, current knowledge of the research and clinical literature, and educational preparation.

_____   3. The strongest empirical knowledge available generated from the synthesis of quality health studies to address a practice problem.

_____   4. Rigorous, explicit clinical standards developed based on the best research evidence available in that area.

_____ 5. Careful examination of all aspects of a study to judge its strengths, limitations, credibility, meaning, and significance.

Synthesizing Research Evidence

Directions: Match each term below with its correct definition. Each term is used only once and all terms are defined.

Terms

a. Meta-analysis
b. Meta-synthesis
c. Mixed-methods systematic review
d. Research syntheses
e. Systematic review

Definitions

_____ 1. Structured, comprehensive synthesis of quantitative studies and meta-analyses in a particular healthcare area to determine the best research evidence available for expert clinicians to use to promote evidence-based practice.

_____ 2. Synthesis or pooling of the results from several previous studies using statistical analyses to determine the effect of an intervention or the strength of a relationship.

_____ 3. Complex, highly structured processes that are best conducted by two or more researchers and expert healthcare clinicians to determine current knowledge for practice.

_____ 4. Systematic synthesis of the findings from independent studies conducted with a variety of methods (quantitative, qualitative, and mixed methods) to determine the current knowledge in an area.

_____ 5. Systematic compiling and integration of qualitative studies to expand understanding and develop a unique interpretation of the studies' findings in a selected area.

EXERCISE 2: LINKING IDEAS

How Research Influences Practice

Directions: The knowledge generated through research is essential to provide a scientific basis for the description, explanation, prediction, and control of nursing practice. Write a definition and provide an example of these four terms.

1. Description:_____

_____

_____

Example:_____

_____

_____

2. Explanation:_____

_____

_____

Example:_____

_____

_____

3. Prediction:_____

_____

_____

Example:_____

_____

_____

4. Control:_____

_____

_____

Example:_____

_____

_____

Historical Events Influencing Nursing Research

Directions: Fill in the blanks with the appropriate word(s) or numbers.

1. _____ is considered the first nurse researcher.

2. The first research journal published in nursing was _____, which is still considered one of the strongest research journals in the profession.

3. Identify three nursing research journals that you might read to keep current in research findings.

   a. _____

   b. _____

   c. _____

4. Many national and international research conferences have been sponsored by _____ _____, the International Honor Society for Nursing, to communicate study findings.

5. The National Center for Nursing Research (NCNR) was established in the year _____ by the National Institutes of Health to promote the funding and conduct of nursing research.

6. The NCNR is now called the _____.

7. _____ is focused on the development, refinement, and use of nursing diagnoses in practice.

8. The national agency that promotes the development and implantation of evidence-based guideline for use in practice is_____

9. The Department of Health and Human Services (DHHS) published _____ to increase the visibility of and identify priorities for health-promotion research.

10. What agency implemented the Magnet Hospital Designation Program® for Excellence in Nursing Services?
_____

Acquiring Knowledge in Nursing

Directions: Fill in the blanks with the appropriate responses.

1. List five ways of acquiring knowledge in nursing, and provide an example of each.

    a. _____

    b. _____

    c. _____

    d. _____

    e. _____

2. Benner's 1984 book, *From Novice to Expert: Excellence and Power in Clinical Practice*, describes the importance of _____ in acquiring nursing knowledge.

3. Identify Benner's five levels of experience in the development of clinical knowledge and expertise that are relevant today.

    a. _____

    b. _____

    c. _____

    d. _____

    e. _____

4. _____ knowledge provides an evidence base for the description, explanation, prediction, and control of nursing practice.

5. A "gut feeling" or "hunch" is an example of _____, which nurses have found useful in identifying patients' changes in health status.

6. What type of reasoning is used in the following example? _____

   Human beings experience pain.
   Babies are human beings.
   Therefore, babies experience pain.

7. Identify three important outcomes that might be examined with outcomes research.

   a. _____

   b. _____

   c. _____

8. Sethares and Asselin (2017) conducted a study to determine the effects of guided reflection on the self-care maintenance and management of patients with heart failure (HF). Review this study in the Research Article Library on
   the Evolve website for *Understanding Nursing Research*, 7th edition, at http://evolve.elsevier.com/grove/
   understanding. What type of research methodology was implemented in conducting this study?
   _____

   Provide a rationale for your answer: _____
   _____
   _____

Linking Research Methods to Types of Research

Directions: Match the following research methods with the specific type of research. One type of research includes both
quantitative and qualitative research methods.

Research Methods
a. Qualitative research method
b. Quantitative research method

Types of Research

_____   1. Correlational research

_____   2. Descriptive research

_____   3. Ethnographic research

_____   4. Experimental research

_____   5. Exploratory-descriptive qualitative research

_____   6. Grounded theory research

_____   7. Phenomenological research

_____   8. Quasi-experimental research

_____   9. Mixed methods research

Nurses' Roles in Research

Directions: Match the levels of nurses' educational preparation with the research activities that each group of nurses is **primarily** responsible for according to the guidelines of the American Nurses Association (ANA) and American Association of Colleges of Nursing (AACN). More than one nurses' educational preparation may be selected for some of the activities.

Nurses' Educational Preparation

a. Bachelor of Science in Nursing (BSN)
b. Master of Science in Nursing (MSN)
c. Doctorate of Nursing Practice (DNP)
d. Doctorate of Philosophy (PhD) in Nursing
e. Postdoctorate

Research Activities

_____ 1. Uses research evidence in practice with guidance.

_____ 2. Develops and coordinates funded research programs.

_____ 3. Critically appraises studies.

_____ 4. Develops nursing knowledge through research and theory development.

_____ 5. Participates in the development of evidence-based guidelines.

_____ 6. Assists in conducting research projects.

_____ 7. Conducts independent research projects.

_____ 8. Critically appraises studies and synthesizes research evidence to develop and refine protocols and policies for a selected healthcare agency.

_____ 9. Mentors PhD-prepared researchers.

_____ 10. Coordinates research teams of BSN-, MSN-, and DNP-prepared nurses.

Determining the Strength of Levels of Research Evidence

Directions: List the following examples of research evidence in numeric order from 1 representing the strongest or best evidence to 6 representing the weakest evidence.

_____ Single correlational study examining the relationships of body mass index, hours watching television per week, and hours on the computer each day.

_____ Systematic review used to develop the evidence-based guidelines for diagnosis and management of hypertension.

_____ Mixed methods systematic review of qualitative and quantitative studies about effectiveness of medication administration technologies on medication errors.

_____ Meta-analysis of experimental studies (randomized controlled trials [RCT]) and quasi-experimental studies to examine interventions to reduce the weight of obese school-age children.

_____ Opinions of respected authorities on the management of diabetes.

_____ Single qualitative study of the process of weaning older adult patients from mechanical ventilation.

EXERCISE 3: WEB-BASED INFORMATION AND RESOURCES

Directions: Answer the following questions with the appropriate website or relevant information.

1. Identify the current mission of the National Institute of Nursing Research (NINR). Search the NINR website for this information.

   _____

   _____

   _____

2. The Agency for Healthcare Research and Quality (AHRQ) has an excellent website that includes evidence-based practice guidelines at _____.

3. Identify the website for the 2014 evidence-based guidelines for the management of hypertension (HTN) in adults:
   _____

4. Identify the website for *Healthy People 2020*: _____

5. On the *Healthy People 2020* website, identify the page for Topics and Objectives on Adolescent Health:
   _____

6. Identify the website for Quality and Safety Education for Nurses (QSEN) competencies for pre-licensure nursing education: _____

7. Search the QSEN prelicensure nursing education website for the Evidence-Based Practice (EBP) Competency and identify this competency: _____
   _____

   Also review the knowledge, skills, and attitudes (KSAs) listed for the EBP Competency.

EXERCISE 4: CONDUCTING CRITICAL APPRAISALS TO BUILD AN EVIDENCE-BASED PRACTICE

Directions: Locate the research articles (listed below) in Appendices A, B, and C. Review the titles, abstracts, and authors' credentials for these three articles. Identify the type of research conducted in each study.

Research Methods
a. Mixed methods research method
b. Qualitative research method
c. Quantitative research method

Articles

_____ 1. Hallas, D., Koslap-Petraco, M., & Fletcher, J. (2017). Social-emotional development of toddlers: Randomized controlled trial of an office-based intervention. *Journal of Pediatric Nursing, 33*(1), 33–40. (Provided in Appendix A)

_____ 2. Erikson, A., & Davies, B. (2017). Maintaining integrity: How nurses navigate boundaries in pediatric palliative care. *Journal of Pediatric Nursing, 35*(1), 42–49. (Provided in Appendix B)

_____ 3. Wendler, M. C., Smith, K., Ellenburg, W., Gill, R., Anderson, L., & Spiegel-Thayer, K. (2017). "To see with my own eyes": Experiences of family visits during phase 1 recovery. *Journal of PeriAnesthesia Nursing, 32*(1), 45–57. (Provided in Appendix C)

Researchers' Credentials

Directions: Review the educational, research, and clinical credentials of the authors of the three research articles in Appendices A, B, and C. The articles include some information about the authors, but you can also search for the authors' credentials and accomplishments online.

1. Discuss whether Hallas et al. (2017) have the educational, research, and clinical preparation to conduct their study.

_____

_____

_____

_____

_____

_____

_____

_____

2. Discuss whether Erikson and Davies (2017) have the educational, research, and clinical preparation to conduct their study.

_____

_____

_____

_____

_____

_____

3. Discuss whether Wendler et al. (2017) have the educational, research, and clinical preparation to conduct their study.

_____

_____

_____

_____

_____

_____

_____

Study Titles and Abstracts

Directions: Critical appraisal of the title and abstract of the Hallas et al. (2017) study.

1. Critical appraisal of the title of the Hallas et al. (2017) study: _____

_____

_____

_____

2. Critical appraisal of the abstract of the Hallas et al. (2017) study: _____

_____

_____

_____

_____

Directions: Post your ideas for the following on your Research Course Discussion Board. Look for input from other students and faculty.

1. Critical appraisal of the title and abstract for the Erikson and Davies (2017) study.

2. Critical appraisal of the title and abstract for the Wendler et al. (2017) study.

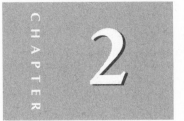

Introduction to Quantitative Research

CHAPTER 2

INTRODUCTION

You need to read Chapter 2 and then complete the following exercises. These exercises will assist you in learning the steps of the quantitative research process; identifying the different types of quantitative research (descriptive, correlational, quasi-experimental, and experimental) in the nursing literature; and reading quantitative research reports. The answers for the following exercises are in the Answer Key at the back of the book.

EXERCISE 1: TERMS AND DEFINITIONS

Directions: Match each term below with its correct definition. Each term is used only once and all terms are defined.

Terms

a. Applied or clinical research
b. Assumptions
c. Basic research
d. Control
e. Correlational research
f. Descriptive research
g. Design
h. Generalization
i. Interpretation of research outcomes
j. Limitations

k. Pilot study
l. Quantitative research
m. Quasi-experimental research
n. Reading a research report
o. Research framework
p. Research problem
q. Research purpose
r. Sampling
s. Setting
t. Variables

Definitions

_____ 1. Formal, objective, rigorous, systematic process for generating numerical information about the world that describes, tests relationships, and examines cause-and-effect interactions among variables.

_____ 2. Location for conducting research that can be natural, partially controlled, or highly controlled.

_____ 3. Scientific investigations conducted to generate knowledge that will directly influence clinical practice.

_____ 4. Imposing of rules by the researcher to decrease the possibility of error and increase the probability that the study's findings are an accurate reflection of reality.

_____ 5. Process of selecting a group of participants that are representative of the population being studied.

_____ 6. Pure scientific investigations conducted for the pursuit of "knowledge for knowledge's sake" that are sometimes referred to as bench research.

_____ 7. Extension of the implications of the findings from the sample that was studied to the larger population.

_____   8. Smaller version of a proposed study conducted to develop and/or refine the methodology, such as the intervention, measurement methods, or data collection process, to be used in a larger study.

_____   9. The specific goal or focus of a study that directs the remaining steps of the research process.

_____   10. Restrictions in a study methodology and/or research framework that may decrease the credibility and generalizability of the findings.

_____   11. Type of quantitative research that is conducted to examine causal relationships or to determine the effect of an independent variable on the dependent variable, but lacks the control of an experimental study.

_____   12. Use of the skills of skimming, comprehending, and analyzing content from a study.

_____   13. Type of quantitative research that involves the exploration of phenomena in real-life situations.

_____   14. Concepts at various levels of abstraction that are measured, manipulated, or controlled in a study.

_____   15. The abstract, theoretical basis for a study that enables the researcher to link the findings to nursing's body of knowledge.

_____   16. Blueprint for the conduct of a study that maximizes control over factors that could interfere with the study's desired outcome.

_____   17. Type of quantitative research that involves the systematic investigation of associations between or among variables.

_____   18. Step in the research process that involves exploring the significance of the findings, forming conclusions, considering implications for nursing, and suggesting further studies.

_____   19. A step in the research process that identifies the gap in nursing knowledge needed for practice and indicates an area for further research.

_____   20. Statements that are taken for granted or are considered true even though they have not been scientifically tested.

EXERCISE 2: LINKING IDEAS

Control in Quantitative Research

Directions: Fill in the blanks with the appropriate word(s).

1. An experimental study is conducted in a(n) _____ setting.

2. _____ and _____ studies are usually conducted in natural settings and are not controlled to the same degree as other types of quantitative research.

3. Extraneous variables need to be controlled in _____ and _____ _____ types of quantitative research to ensure that the findings are accurate and not the result of bias or errors.

4. _____ studies should include random assignment of study participants to the intervention and control groups.

5. Frequently, a(n) _____ sampling method is used in descriptive and correlational studies. However, a(n) _____ sampling method might also be used.

6. A study participant's home is an example of a(n) _____ setting.

7. Laboratories, research units, and research centers are examples of _____ settings where experimental research is conducted.

8. Researcher control is greatest in what type of quantitative research? _____

9. Hospital units are examples of _____ settings that allow the researchers to control some of the extraneous variables in the study.

10. Quantitative studies that include interventions are _____.

Steps of the Research Process

Directions: Fill in the blanks with the appropriate word(s).

1. The research process is similar to the _____ and the _____ process.

2. List the steps of the quantitative research process in their typical order of occurrence.

   Step 1_____

   Step 2_____

   Step 3_____

   Step 4_____

   Step 5_____

   Step 6_____

   Step 7_____

   Step 8_____

   Step 9_____

   Step 10_____

   Step 11_____

3. Identify three common assumptions on which various nursing studies have been based.

   a. _____

   b. _____

   c. _____

4. Identify four reasons for conducting a pilot study.

   a. _____

   b. _____

   c. _____

   d. _____

5. Wendler et al. (2017, p. 56) reported: "Generalizability of the study is hampered by the lack of control group, and a convenience sample was used." In a research report, these are examples of _____.

Reading Research Reports

Directions: Fill in the blanks with the appropriate responses.

1. The most common sources for nursing research reports are professional journals. Identify three nursing research journals.

   a. _____

   b. _____

   c. _____

2. Identify two clinical journals that include several research articles in each issue.

   a. _____

   b. _____

3. Identify the four major or primary sections of a research report.

   a. _____

   b. _____

   c. _____

   d. _____

4. Identify four elements or steps of the quantitative research process that are included in the methods section of a research report.

   a. _____

   b. _____

   c. _____

   d. _____

5. The discussion section ties the other sections of the research report together and gives them meaning. Identify five elements or steps that are included in this section of a research report.

   a. _____

   b. _____

   c. _____

   d. _____

   e. _____

6. The problem and purpose are often identified in the _____ section of a research report.

7. The reference list at the end of a research report includes the relevant _____ and _____ sources that provide a basis for the study and are cited in the report.

8. Reading a research report involves _____, _____, and _____ the content of the report.

9. In reading a research report, the comprehending step involves _____

   _____.

10. In reading a research report, the analyzing step involves _____

    _____.

Types of Quantitative Research

Directions: Match the type of quantitative research listed below with the examples of study titles. The types of quantitative research are used more than once.

Type of Quantitative Research
a. Descriptive research
b. Correlational research
c. Quasi-experimental research
d. Experimental research

Examples of Study Titles

_____ 1. Determining the effects of a relaxation technique versus standard care on patients' postoperative pain and anxiety levels in a day surgery center.

_____ 2. Determining the risk behaviors of adolescents and young adults for sexually transmitted diseases.

_____ 3. Examining the associations among age, gender, knowledge of AIDS, and use of condoms by college students.

_____ 4. Comparing the immunization rates in family medicine clinics versus pediatric clinics.

_____ 5. Determining the effect of acupressure on fatigue of female nurses with chronic back pain.

_____ 6. Examining the effect of impaired physical mobility on skeletal muscle atrophy in laboratory rats.

_____ 7. Examining the relationships among hardiness, depression, and coping in institutionalized older adults.

_____ 8. Determining the stress levels and quality of life of family caregivers of older adults with Alzheimer's disease.

_____ 9. Examining the effects of thermal applications on the abdominal temperatures of laboratory dogs.

_____ 10. Examining the relationships among the lipid values, blood pressure, weight, and stress levels of adolescents.

_____ 11. Determining the effect of warm and cold applications on the resolution of intravenous (IV) infiltrations in hospitalized patients.

_____ 12. Comparing the ages and coping skills of mothers pregnant with their first child in three racial groups (White, Black, and Asian/Pacific Islander).

_____ 13. Examining the effects of a preadmission self-instruction program on patients' postoperative activity levels, anxiety levels, pain perception, lengths of hospital stay, and time until return to work.

_____ 14. Using age, nutritional intake, mobility level, weight, level of cognitive function, and serum albumin to predict the risk for pressure ulcers in hospitalized patients on a medical–surgical unit.

_____ 15. Determining the effectiveness of an automated reorientation intervention on delirium prevention in critically ill adults.

EXERCISE 3: WEB-BASED INFORMATION AND RESOURCES

Directions: Search for quantitative study information.

1. During recent years, extensive basic or bench research has been conducted in the United States to describe human genetics. Identify the national organization focused on this research: _____

   _____

   Identify the website for this national organization: _____

   _____

   Identify the website for funding provided by this organization: _____

   _____

   Genomic research began with what project? _____

   _____

2. Identify the website for the National Institute of Nursing Research (NINR): _____
   Search this web page and examine the types of research being conducted in nursing. Review the "Research Highlights" at what NINR web page and identify one on this page. _____

3. Identify the website that presents the findings and reports of the studies funded by the Agency for Healthcare Research and Quality (AHRQ): _____

_____

EXERCISE 4: CONDUCTING CRITICAL APPRAISALS TO BUILD AN EVIDENCE-BASED PRACTICE

Directions: Read the research articles in Appendices A, B, and C and answer the following questions.

Type of Quantitative and/or Qualitative Research

Directions: Identify the type of quantitative and/or qualitative research conducted in each study.

Type of Research

a. Descriptive research
b. Correlational research
c. Quasi-experimental research
d. Experimental research

e. Phenomenological research
f. Grounded theory research
g. Exploratory-descriptive research
h. Ethnographic research

Study

_____ 1. Hallas, D., Koslap-Petraco, M., & Fletcher, J. (2017). Social-emotional development of toddlers: Randomized controlled trial of an office-based intervention. *Journal of Pediatric Nursing, 33*(1), 33–40. (Provided in Appendix A)

_____ 2. Erikson, A., & Davies, B. (2017). Maintaining integrity: How nurses navigate boundaries in pediatric palliative care. *Journal of Pediatric Nursing, 35*(1), 42–49. (Provided in Appendix B)

_____ 3. Wendler, M. C., Smith, K., Ellenburg, W., Gill, R., Anderson, L., & Spiegel-Thayer, K. (2017). "To see with my own eyes": Experiences of family visits during phase 1 recovery. *Journal of PeriAnesthesia Nursing, 32*(1), 45–57. (Provided in Appendix C)

Type of Setting

Directions: Identify the type of setting for each study and provide rationales for your answers.

a. Natural setting
b. Partially controlled setting
c. Highly controlled setting

_____ 1. Hallas et al. (2017) study setting

Rationale: _____

_____

_____

_____

_____   2. Erikson and Davies (2017) study setting

Rationale: _____

_____

_____

_____

_____   3. Wendler et al. (2017) study setting

Rationale: _____

_____

_____

_____

Type of Research Conducted (Applied or Basic)

Directions: Indicate the type of nursing research conducted in each study.

Type of Nursing Research

a. Applied nursing research
b. Basic nursing research

Study

_____   1. Hallas et al. (2017) study

_____   2. Wendler et al. (2017) study

CHAPTER 3

Introduction to Qualitative Research

INTRODUCTION

Read Chapter 3 and then complete the following exercises. These exercises will assist you in learning key terms and reading, comprehending, and critically appraising published qualitative studies. The answers for the following exercises are in the Answer Key at the back of the book.

EXERCISE 1: TERMS AND DEFINITIONS

Directions: Match each term below with its correct definition. Each term is used only once and all terms are defined.

Definitions Related to Qualitative Research
Terms

a. Audit trail
b. Bracketing
c. Dwelling with the data
d. Ethnographic research
e. Ethnonursing research
f. Exploratory-descriptive qualitative research
g. Field notes
h. Focus group
i. Grounded theory research

j. Methodological congruence
k. Moderator or facilitator
l. Participant
m. Phenomena
n. Phenomenological research
o. Rigor
p. Transcription
q. Triangulation
r. Unstructured interview

Definitions

_____ 1. Research based on a pragmatic philosophy and focused on increasing understanding or finding a solution.

_____ 2. Typing a verbatim narrative from a recorded interview or focus group.

_____ 3. A person selected to guide the discussion of a focus group and may share characteristics of focus-group members.

_____ 4. Questioning research participants orally without a fixed set of questions.

_____ 5. A record of decisions made during data collection, analysis, and interpretation.

_____ 6. When the data collection and other methods are consistent with the research problem and study purpose.

_____ 7. Characteristics of study methods indicate the strength and credibility of a qualitative study.

_____ 8. Gathering data from multiple participants simultaneously to encourage interaction and discussion.

_____ 9. Studies focused on the lived experience.

_____ 10. Using Dr. Leininger's methods to describe a cultural group.

_____ 11. Setting aside one's values and perspectives during the data collection and analysis process.

_____ 12. Qualitative method that describes social processes and proposes a framework of related concepts.

_____ 13. Collecting data from two or more perspectives for the purpose of describing a unique perspective where they converge.

_____ 14. Notes from a research observation.

_____ 15. Researcher spends considerable periods of time reading and reflecting on the data.

_____ 16. A person from whom data are collected during a qualitative study.

_____ 17. Conscious awareness of experiences that comprise being alive.

_____ 18. Study of cultures based on anthropology.

Definitions Related to Ethnography
Terms
a. Critical ethnography
b. Emic approach
c. Etic approach
d. Focused ethnography
e. Going native
f. Immersed
g. Key informant

Definitions

_____ 1. Type of study that explores the culture of a specific group of people or an organization for a shorter period of time.

_____ 2. Gaining familiarity with the aspects of a culture by spending time in it.

_____ 3. A person with extensive knowledge and influence in a culture who may facilitate the work of an ethnographer.

_____ 4. A researcher becomes a part of the culture and loses the ability to objectively observe.

_____ 5. Studying a culture using an insider perspective that recognizes the uniqueness of the individual.

_____ 6. Type of study that examines the political and socio-ecological factors of a culture.

_____ 7. Studying a culture using the perspective of a naive outsider.

Definitions in Your Own Words

Directions: Define the following terms in your own words without looking at your textbook. Then check your definitions with those in the glossary of your textbook. Using this strategy, you can identify elements of the term that are not yet clear in your mind. Reread that section of the chapter to clarify your understanding of the term.

1. Observation: _____

_____

2. Coding: _____

_____

3. Researcher-participant relationship: _____

_____

EXERCISE 2: LINKING IDEAS

People and Their Contributions to Qualitative Research

Directions: Match the names of people below with the correct description. Each name is used only once and all people are described.

Description

a. Philosopher associated with the interpretive approach to phenomenology
b. Developed the Sunshine Model of Transcultural Nursing Care
c. Philosopher associated with the descriptive approach to phenomenology
d. Person who developed the symbolic interaction theory
e. Their early studies on dying led to the grounded theory method

Names

_____ 1. Leininger

_____ 2. Glaser and Strauss

_____ 3. Husserl

_____ 4. Heidegger

_____ 5. Mead

Qualitative Research Methodology

Directions: Fill in the blanks with the appropriate word(s).

1. During a phenomenological study, the researcher listens to the recordings of interviews several times and reads and rereads the transcripts to _____ with the data.

2. An ethnographer lives in a different culture for a year, learns the language, and slowly stops communicating with family and friends in her home country. When asked when she plans to return, the ethnographer says she has not decided because she prefers the culture here more than she does the culture of her own country. There is a danger that the ethnographer has "gone _____."

3. The observer writes down comments and descriptions of body language during the focus group. The observer is preparing _____.

4. During a grounded theory study of men living with chronic illness, the researcher continues to recruit participants until _____ is reached, defined as additional participants not providing new information.

5. The researcher begins unstructured interviews with a general question to allow participants to tell their experiences of being diagnosed with stomach cancer. If a participant stops talking and seems unable to continue, the researcher has prepared short questions to help the participant continue or add new information. These questions are called _____.

Approaches to Qualitative Research

Directions: Match each qualitative approach with its characteristics. Label them P, G, E, and/or ED according to the key below for each area. All answers will be used once. All answers will be used once and some more than once.

Qualitative Approach

P = Phenomenological research
G = Grounded theory research

E = Ethnographic research
EDQ = Exploratory-descriptive qualitative research

Characteristics

_____   1. May use key informants in the study of cultures.

_____   2. Refers to a philosophy and a research method.

_____   3. Often based on a pragmatic philosophy.

_____   4. Seeks to develop a framework of concepts or theory.

_____   5. Emerged from the discipline of anthropology.

_____   6. Undertaken to solve a problem or obtain information to use to improve a service.

_____   7. Studies the meaning of a lived experience.

_____   8. Interested in the social processes.

EXERCISE 3: WEB-BASED INFORMATION AND RESOURCES

1. What are the differences between quantitative and qualitative research? Find websites that provide comparisons of quantitative and qualitative research. Provide at least one URL below.

_____

Directions: Use the websites you find to complete the table with differences in quantitative and qualitative research for each aspect of the research.

	Qualitative	Quantitative
Data		
How will findings be used?		
Perspective		
Characteristics of rigor		

	Qualitative	Quantitative
Methods		
Size of sample		
Relationship between researcher and participants		

2. What can you learn about a qualitative study from reading the title and the introduction and skimming the article? To answer this question, go to the Research Article Library on the Evolve website for *Understanding Nursing Research*, 7th edition, at http://evolve.elsevier.com/grove/understanding, and find the qualitative study conducted by Chin (2017).

    Chin, E. (2017). The COPD exacerbation experience: A qualitative description. *Applied Nursing Research, 38*(1), 38–44.

    Directions: Read the title and the introduction, skim the article, and complete the following information.

Study Characteristic	Answer
Country/state in which the study was conducted.	
Identify the qualitative approach conducted (phenomenology, grounded theory, exploratory-descriptive qualitative, ethnography research).	
Identify the human experience or topic of the study.	

Describe the sample, including the total number, gender, reason for hospitalization, mean age, and ethnicity of the majority of the participants.	
How were the data collected?	

EXERCISE 4: CONDUCTING CRITICAL APPRAISALS TO BUILD AN EVIDENCE-BASED PRACTICE

Directions: Read the Erikson and Davies (2017) article in Appendix B of this study guide. Answer the following questions about that qualitative study.

1. What was the purpose of the study? _____

   _____

   _____

2. Which qualitative method was conducted in this study? How did the method fit with the purpose of the study?

   _____

   _____

   _____

3. What was the overall theme that was identified by Erikson and Davies (2017)? _____

   _____

4. Table 1 in the article displays information about the participants. Use information in the table to answer the following questions.

   a. How many of the nurses worked at the children's hospital? _____

   b. What was the average years of nursing experience? _____

   c. How many participants were Black? _____

5. How were the data collected? _____

   _____

6. Were the interview questions relevant for the study purpose? Explain your answer.

   _____

   _____

7. Were the data analysis and interpretation processes consistent with the philosophical orientation, research problem, and purpose of the study? Provide a rationale for your answer.

   _____

   _____

   _____

   _____

   _____

   _____

8. Did the researcher provide evidence of the themes by including exemplar quotations? Provide an example for your answer.

   _____

   _____

   _____

   _____

   _____

   _____

9. Review Figure 1 and the caption under the figure to answer the following questions.
   a. What two types of boundaries form the outer solid circle? _____

   _____

   b. Near the top of the figure, there is the label "Mitigating the tension." What two competing aspects of the nursing role create the tension? _____

   _____

c.   Erikson and Davies (2017) identify three ways to "take care of self." List the three ways they identified.

1). _____

2). _____

3). _____

Directions: Read the Wendler et al. (2017) article in Appendix C of this study guide. Answer the following questions about the qualitative component of the mixed methods study. Chapter 14 includes additional critical appraisal questions about the Wendler et al. (2017) study.

10.   How were the qualitative data collected for this study?

_____

_____

_____

11.   The researchers used open coding and in vivo coding during the initial analysis of the qualitative data. How many secondary codes were created through constant comparison? _____ How many categories remained after the final data reduction? _____

12.   Review Table 4. Provide one category with an example used to support the category.

_____

_____

_____

_____

_____

Examining Ethics in Nursing Research

INTRODUCTION

You need to read Chapter 4 and then complete the following exercises. These exercises will assist you in understanding and critically appraising the ethical aspects of a variety of nursing studies. The answers for these exercises are in the Answer Key at the back of the book.

EXERCISE 1: TERMS AND DEFINITIONS

Directions: Match each term below with its correct definition. Each term is used only once and all terms are defined.

Terms

a. Anonymity
b. Autonomy
c. Benefit–risk ratio
d. Confidentiality
e. Deception
f. Discomfort and harm
g. Ethical principles
h. Identifiable private information (IPI)
i. Informed consent
j. Institutional review board (IRB)
k. Nontherapeutic research
l. Plagiarism
m. Privacy
n. Research misconduct
o. Therapeutic research

Definitions

_____ 1. Anticipated or actual physical, emotional, social, or economic risks associated with a study.

_____ 2. Condition in which a subject's identity cannot be linked, even by the researcher, with his or her individual responses.

_____ 3. Agreement by a prospective subject to participate voluntarily in a study after he or she has indicated understanding of the essential information about the study.

_____ 4. Research conducted to generate knowledge for a discipline; the results might benefit future patients, but will probably not benefit the research subjects.

_____ 5. A committee of peers that approves, disapproves, or requests changes to a study after examining a study for ethical concerns.

_____ 6. The act of misleading subjects which is only permissible if there is no long-term harm and subjects consent to participation with the knowledge that they will be unaware or misled about an aspect of the study.

_____ 7. Freedom of an individual to determine the time, extent, and general circumstances under which private information will be shared with or withheld from others.

    _____   8.   The balance between potential benefits and risks in a study that must be weighed by researchers to promote the conduct of ethical research.

    _____   9.   Research that provides a patient with an opportunity to receive an experimental treatment that might have beneficial results.

    _____   10.   Principles of respect for persons, beneficence, and justice, which are relevant to the conduct of research.

    _____   11.   Management of private data in research in such a way that subjects' identities are not linked with their responses.

    _____   12.   Practices such as fabrication, falsification, or forging of data; dishonest manipulation of the study design or methods; and plagiarism.

    _____   13.   Any information, including demographic information, collected from an individual that is created or received by healthcare providers, health plan, or healthcare clearinghouse.

    _____   14.   A person's freedom to conduct their life as they choose, without external controls.

    _____   15.   The appropriation of another person's ideas, processes, results, or words without giving appropriate credit, including those obtained through confidential review of others' research proposals and manuscripts.

EXERCISE 2: LINKING IDEAS

Directions: Fill in the blanks with the appropriate responses.

1.   List the four elements of the research informed consent process.

    a.   _____

    b.   _____

    c.   _____

    d.   _____

2.   Identify five general information requirements that are included in a comprehensive study consent form.

    a.   _____

    b.   _____

    c.   _____

    d.   _____

    e.   _____

3.   _____ consent means that prospective adults with heart failure have decided to take part in the study of their own volition, without coercion or any undue influence, to improve their management of a chronic illness.

4.   Study participants with _____ (e.g., the mentally ill, cognitively impaired, or children) are vulnerable and incompetent to consent to participate in research.

5. A study conducted by a student must be reviewed by their university faculty and also the _____ _____ of the university and the agency where data will be collected.

6. The three levels of institutional review of research are:

   a. _____

   b. _____

   c. _____

7. During a presentation of study findings, a researcher inadvertently shows raw data, which includes subjects' names and presence or absence of drug use by the subjects. This error is an example of a _____ _____. Provide a rationale for your answer. _____

   _____

   _____

   _____

   _____

8. Who determines the level of institutional review for a study? _____

   _____

9. A study that involved examining the effects of a new drug on patients' serum lipid values would probably require what type of institutional review? _____

10. Identify three possible types of research misconduct.

    a. _____

    b. _____

    c. _____

11. The _____ is a federal agency that was organized for reporting and investigating research misconduct.

12. Is research misconduct present in nursing? (**Yes** or **No**) Provide a rationale for your answer.

    _____

    _____

    _____

13. Are animals used in research conducted by nurses? (**Yes** or **No**) Provide a rationale for your answer.

    _____

    _____

    _____

14. What federal office was instituted to protect the welfare of animals used in research? _____

_____

15. What organization was developed to ensure the humane treatment of animals in research and who grants accreditation to many institutions?

_____

_____

Historical Events, Ethical Codes, and Regulations

Directions: Match each unethical study listed below with the correct description. You will use all answers more than once.

Unethical Study

a. Jewish Chronic Disease Hospital Study
b. Nazi Medical Experiments
c. Tuskegee Syphilis Study
d. Willowbrook Study

Description

_____ 1. Subjects were exposed to freezing temperatures, high altitudes, poisons, untested drugs, infections and surgeries without anesthesia.

_____ 2. The study was conducted to determine the natural course of syphilis in Black men.

_____ 3. Subjects were deliberately infected with the hepatitis virus in this study.

_____ 4. Subjects commonly sustained permanent physical damage or were killed.

_____ 5. Subjects did not receive penicillin when it was identified during the course of the study as an effective treatment for their disease.

_____ 6. The purpose of this study was to determine the patients' rejection responses to live cancer cells.

_____ 7. The subjects in this study were institutionalized mentally retarded children.

_____ 8. The Nuremberg Code was developed in response to these unethical experiments.

_____ 9. Subjects and physicians providing care for the subjects were unaware that the study was being conducted.

_____ 10. The National Commission for the Protection of Human Subjects of Biomedical and Behavioral Research was formed in response to the public outcry over this study.

Ethical Principles

Directions: Match the ethical principle with the example from research. You will use some answers more than once and some examples might address more than one ethical principle.

Ethical Principle

a. Principle of beneficence
b. Principle of justice
c. Principle of respect for persons

Example

_____ 1. The 7- to 16-year-old subjects of a study were given the right to assent to participate in the study.

_____ 2. The researcher developed a therapeutic study that would benefit the study subjects.

_____ 3. The subjects involved in a study at a clinic where they receive care were reassured of their right to withdraw from the study at any time and that their care at the clinic would not be affected by withdrawal from the study.

_____ 4. The researcher carefully selected study inclusion and exclusion criteria based on scientific evidence and logical considerations and obtained a study sample that fairly represented the demographic characteristics of the target population.

_____ 5. The researcher carefully considered risks and benefits in the development of a study to reduce the risk to potential subjects.

Federal Regulations Influencing the Conduct of Research

Directions: Match the federal regulation with the content or definitions provided. You will use some answers more than once.

Federal Regulation

a. US Department of Health and Human Services (DHHS) Protection of Human Subjects Regulations (Common Rule)
b. US Food and Drug Administration (FDA) Protection of Human Subjects Regulations
c. Health Insurance Portability and Accountability Act (HIPAA)

Content or Definition

_____ 1. Regulations provide direction for conducting research with vulnerable populations such as children and prisoners.

_____ 2. Regulations were developed to protect identifiable private information (IPI).

_____ 3. Regulations were developed in response to the Belmont Report and are part of the Code of Federal Regulations (CFR).

_____ 4. Regulations are focused on clinical trials to generate new drugs and refine existing drug treatments.

_____ 5. Regulations that apply to broader situations than research of human subjects.

Ethics of Published Studies

Directions: Match each ethical term with the appropriate example from a published study. You can read these studies in the study guide appendices or in the Research Article Library on the Evolve website for *Understanding Nursing Research*, 7th edition, at http://evolve.elsevier.com/grove/understanding.

Ethical Term

a. Assent
b. Coercion
c. Consent
d. Deception
e. Institutional review board (IRB)
f. Vulnerable population

Examples of Ethical Content From Published Studies

_____ 1. Chin's (2017, p. 39) qualitative study was approved by the "researcher's university, as well as at the hospitals in which recruitment and data collection occurred." These are examples of what type of approvals?

_____ 2. "Participants with COPD were referred to the researcher by the resource RN of each unit after obtaining permission from the patient for the researcher to meet with them" (Chin, 2017, p. 39). What is obtaining permission prior to contact with the researcher a safeguard against?

_____ 3. Hallas, Koslap-Petraco, and Fletcher (2017) conducted a randomized controlled trial with mother and toddler subjects. In research, toddlers are an example of what type of subject?

_____ 4. Both adult and child participants were included in the Hallas et al. (2017) study. What is the informed agreement to participate in research from an adult participant referred to as? What is agreement to participate in research from a child referred to as?

_____ 5. Coleman (2017, p. 139) conducted a descriptive correlational study in which "The participants were provided an overview of the purpose of the study including: procedures, risks and benefits." The information provided to potential subjects by Coleman (2017) is an important safeguard against what type of risk?

EXERCISE 3: WEB-BASED INFORMATION AND RESOURCES

Directions: Fill in the blanks with the appropriate websites.

1. Identify the website for the US Department of Health and Human Services (US DHHS, 2016) federal regulations for the protection of human subjects in research, which is also referred to as the "Common Rule."

_____

   Review these regulations to determine how human subjects are protected during the conduct of research.

2. The ethical principles of respect for persons, beneficence, and justice were developed as part of the Belmont Report that guided the development of the DHHS regulations for the protection of human subjects in research. Locate the Belmont Report online:

_____

   Review the focus of these three ethical principles.

3. Identify the website for the US Food and Drug Administration (US FDA, 2017) regulations for the protection of human subjects:

_____

4. Locate the website of the HIPAA Privacy Rule that is focused on the information needed by researchers:

_____

   Review this information to determine how researchers protect study participants' private information.

5. Locate the website for the Office of Research Integrity (ORI), where the case summaries of research misconduct are discussed:

_____

Review some of the case summaries and identify what types of research misconduct occurred.

6. Identify the website for the Office of Laboratory Animal Welfare (OLAW): _____

_____

Review the policies regarding the humane treatment of animals by researchers and institutions.

EXERCISE 4: CONDUCTING CRITICAL APPRAISALS TO BUILD AN EVIDENCE-BASED PRACTICE

Directions: Review the research articles in Appendices A, B, and C to answer the following questions.

1. Is the Hallas et al. (2017) study ethical? Use the critical appraisal guidelines for ethical aspects of the study presented in Chapter 4 of *Understanding Nursing Research*, 7th edition.

_____

_____

_____

_____

_____

_____

_____

_____

_____

_____

_____

2. Is the Erikson and Davies (2017) study ethical? Use the critical appraisal guidelines for ethical aspects of the study presented in Chapter 4 of *Understanding Nursing Research,* 7th edition.

_____

_____

_____

_____

_____

_____

_____

_____

_____

_____

_____

3. Is the Wendler et al. (2017) study ethical? Use the critical appraisal guidelines for ethical aspects of the study presented in Chapter 4 of *Understanding Nursing Research*, 7th edition.

_____

_____

_____

_____

_____

_____

_____

_____

_____

_____

_____

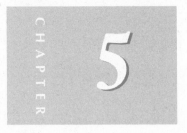

Examining Research Problems, Purposes, and Hypotheses

INTRODUCTION

You need to read Chapter 5 and then complete the following exercises. These exercises will assist you in critically appraising problems, purposes, objectives, questions, hypotheses, and variables in published studies. The answers to these exercises are in the Answer Key at the back of the book.

EXERCISE 1: TERMS AND DEFINITIONS

Directions: Match each term below with its correct definition. Each term is used only once and all terms are defined.

Terms
a. Conceptual definition
b. Demographic variable
c. Dependent variable
d. Extraneous variable
e. Hypothesis
f. Independent variable
g. Operational definition
h. Research problem
i. Research purpose
j. Research question
k. Research topic

Definitions

_____ 1. Description of how variables will be measured in a study, such as measuring acute pain in children with the FACES scale.

_____ 2. Clear, concise statement of the specific goal or focus of a study that is generated from the research problem.

_____ 3. The intervention or treatment that is manipulated or varied by the researcher to create an effect on the dependent variable.

_____ 4. Researchers attempt to identify and control the influence of these variables in quasi-experimental and experimental studies to reduce the potential for error in study findings.

_____ 5. Concise interrogative statement developed to direct a study; focuses on description of variables, examination of relationships among variables, and determination of differences among two or more groups.

_____ 6. Concept or broad problem area, such as self-care deficit, that provides the basis for generating numerous research problems.

_____ 7. Formal statement of the expected relationship or outcome from studying variables in a specified population.

_____ 8. Variables reported in a study to describe the attributes or characteristics of study participants in the sample.

_____ 9. Definition that provides a variable or concept with theoretical meaning that might be obtained from a theory, concept analysis, or qualitative studies.

_____ 10. The response, behavior, or outcome that is predicted or explained in research; changes in this variable are presumed to be caused by the independent variable.

_____ 11. Area of concern or gap in nursing knowledge that requires research.

Types of Hypotheses

Directions: Match each type of hypothesis with the correct definition.

Type of Hypothesis

a. Associative hypothesis
b. Causal hypothesis
c. Complex hypothesis
d. Directional hypothesis

e. Nondirectional hypothesis
f. Null hypothesis
g. Research hypothesis
h. Simple hypothesis

Definitions

_____ 1. Hypothesis stating that no relationships exist among the variables being studied.

_____ 2. Hypothesis stating that a relationship exists but not predicting the exact nature of the relationship.

_____ 3. Hypothesis stating the relationship (associative or causal) between two variables.

_____ 4. Hypothesis stating the specific nature of the interaction or relationship among two or more variables.

_____ 5. Hypothesis stating a relationship between two variables in which one variable (independent variable) is thought to cause or determine the presence of the other variable (dependent variable).

_____ 6. Hypothesis predicting the relationships (associative or causal) among three or more variables.

_____ 7. Alternative hypothesis to the null hypothesis; states that a relationship exists among two or more variables.

_____ 8. Hypothesis stating a relationship in which variables that occur or exist together in the real world are identified; thus when one variable changes, the other variables change.

EXERCISE 2: LINKING IDEAS

Research Problem and Purpose

Directions: Fill in the blanks with the appropriate responses.

1. A clearly stated research purpose includes:

   a. _____,

   b. _____, and usually the

   c. _____.

2. Research problems and purposes are significant if they have the potential to generate and refine relevant knowledge that:

   a. _____

   b. _____

   c. _____

3. Identify two national organizations or agencies that have developed lists of research priorities relevant to nursing.

   a. _____

   b. _____

4. The feasibility of a research problem and purpose is determined by examining the following:

   a. _____

   b. _____

   c. _____

   d. _____

5. A study was funded by the National Institute of Nursing Research (NINR), which documents the _____ of the study.

Understanding Hypotheses

Directions: Ten sample hypotheses are presented in this section. Identify each hypothesis using the terms listed below. Four terms are needed to identify each hypothesis. The correct answer for hypothesis #1 is provided as an example.

Terms

a. Associative hypothesis
b. Causal hypothesis
c. Complex hypothesis
d. Directional hypothesis
e. Nondirectional hypothesis
f. Null hypothesis
g. Research hypothesis
h. Simple hypothesis

Hypotheses

<u>b, c, d, g</u>   1. Relaxation therapy is more effective than standard care in decreasing pain perception and use of pain medications in adults with chronic arthritic pain.

_____   2. Age, family support, and health status are related to the self-care abilities of nursing-home residents.

_____   3. Healthy adults involved in an exercise program have lower low-density lipoprotein (LDL), higher high-density lipoprotein (HDL), and lower cardiovascular risk levels than adults not involved in the program.

_____   4. Quality of life is related to self-care abilities in adults with mental illness.

_____   5. Low-back massage is more effective in decreasing perception of low-back pain than no massage in patients with chronic low-back pain.

_____ 6.   There are no differences in complication rates or incidence of phlebitis between patients in whom heparin locks are changed every 72 hours and those where locks are left in place for up to 168 hours.

_____ 7.   Increased time on the operating table, lower diastolic blood pressure, higher age, and lower preoperative albumin levels are related to the increased development of pressure ulcers in hospitalized older adults.

_____ 8.   Intensive care unit (ICU) patients exposed to an audio tape of a significant family member's voice have less delirium than ICU patients without exposure to an audio tape.

_____ 9.   Nurses' perceived work stress, work position, and years of work experience are related to their perception of burnout in their job.

_____ 10.   Communication of high blood pressure education through a mobile application is no more effective than education provided during a clinic visit on patients' knowledge of high blood pressure.

11.   State hypothesis #2 as a directional hypothesis. _____

_____

_____

12.   State hypothesis #5 as a null hypothesis. _____

_____

_____

Identifying Types of Study Variables

Directions: Match each example variable below with the most likely type of variable that might be included in a study. All the variables will be used more than once.

Type of Variable
a.   Demographic variable
b.   Dependent variable
c.   Independent variable

Example Variables

_____ 1.   Age

_____ 2.   Immunization plan provided by text messaging

_____ 3.   Perception of pain

_____ 4.   Gender

_____ 5.   Length of hospital stay

_____ 6.   Ethnic background

_____ 7.   Anxiety level

_____ 8.   Incidence of deep vein thrombosis

_____ 9.   Educational level

_____ 10.   Low-back massage

_____ 11.   Depression level

_____ 12.   Yoga classes

_____ 13.   Hemoglobin A1c

_____ 14.   Low-density lipoprotein (LDL) value

_____ 15.   Marital status

_____ 16.   DVD on nutrition presented in clinic

Understanding Study Variables

Directions: Match these variables with the examples provided below. Some of the variables will be used more than once.

Terms

a. Demographic variables
b. Dependent variables
c. Extraneous variable
d. Independent variable

Examples

_____ 1. Acute pain is a physiological and psychological response to trauma that is commonly examined in studies.

_____ 2. When researchers examined the effects of nasal oxygen on oral temperature, all patients with fever were excluded from the study because fever had the potential to affect the study's findings. This is an example of what type of variable?

_____ 3. Six-week physical therapy program for the elderly over 70 years of age.

_____ 4. Variables such as age, gender, and medical diagnoses are measured to describe the sample.

_____ 5. Blood pressure reading, pulse, and oxygen saturation level following exercise.

_____ 6. Type 2 diabetes educational program provided through a mobile application on the patients' phone.

EXERCISE 3: WEB-BASED INFORMATION AND RESOURCES

Directions: The following questions require identifying and searching selected websites. Review the key information provided on the websites.

1. The references for the Hallas et al. (2017) study included the Centers for Disease Control and Prevention (CDC). Identify the home page for the CDC:

   _____

2. On the CDC website, search for the topic: "Violence Prevention." Did you find information about child abuse and neglect prevention? **(Yes or No)** Identify the website for this topic:

   _____

   _____

3. Identify the website for the National Institute of Nursing Research (NINR):

   _____

4. According to the NINR, what is nursing research? _____

   _____

   _____

5. Locate the Strohfus, Kim, Palma, Duke, Remington, and Roberts (2017) study in the Research Article Library on the Evolve website for *Understanding Nursing Research*, 7th edition, at http://evolve.elsevier.com/ grove/understanding. This study was focused on improving immunization rates in family medicine and pediatric offices.

   a. Identify a website that details the schedule for providing immunizations to children and adolescents less than 18 years of age: _____

   _____

   b. Identify a website that details the schedule for providing immunizations to adults: _____

   _____

EXERCISE 4: CONDUCTING CRITICAL APPRAISALS TO BUILD AN EVIDENCE-BASED PRACTICE

Problem and Purpose

Hallas, Koslap-Petraco, and Fletcher (2017) Study

Directions: Review the Hallas et al. (2017) research article in Appendix A and answer the following questions.

1. State the problem of this study.

   a. Significance:_____

   _____

   _____

   _____

   _____

   _____

   b. Background:_____

   _____

   _____

   _____

   _____

   c. Hallas et al. (2017, p. 34) reported that "mother–toddler interactions in waiting areas in a pediatric primary care office in which mothers were interacting inappropriately with toddlers escalating challenging toddler behaviors. The mother–toddler interactions were also viewed as impeding the social-emotional development of these toddlers." This comment provided a basis for the following research problem statement: _____

   _____

   _____

   _____

2. State the purpose of this study. _____

_____

_____

_____

_____

3. Are the problem and the purpose significant? (**Yes** or **No**) Provide a rationale for your answer. _____

_____

_____

_____

_____

_____

_____

4. Does the purpose identify the variables, population, and setting for this study? _____

    a. Identify the variables. _____

_____

_____

    b. Identify the population. _____

    c. Identify the setting. _____

5. Is it feasible for the researchers to study the problem and purpose? (**Yes** or **No**) Provide a rationale. _____

_____

_____

_____

_____

_____

Erikson and Davies (2017) Study

Directions: Review the Erikson and Davies (2017) research article in Appendix B and answer the following questions.

1. State the problem of this study.

    a. Significance: _____

_____

_____

_____

_____

b. Background: _____

_____

_____

_____

_____

c. Problem statement: _____

_____

_____

2. State the purpose of this study.

a. Purpose: _____

_____

b. Is this study purpose clearly presented? **(Yes or No)** Provide a rationale for your answer. _____

_____

_____

c. The purpose might have been more clearly stated as: _____

_____

_____

3. Are the problem and the purpose significant? **(Yes** or **No)** Provide a rationale. _____

_____

_____

_____

4. Indicate if the research purpose identified the concepts, population, and/or setting for this study. _____

_____

a. Identify the research concepts. _____

_____

    b.   Identify the population. _____

    c.   Identify the setting. _____

5.   Is it feasible for these researchers to study this problem and purpose? **(Yes or No)** Provide a rationale. _____

_____

_____

_____

_____

_____

Wendler, Smith, Ellenburg, Gill, Anderson, and Spiegel-Thayer (2017) Study

Directions: Review the Wendler et al. (2017) research article in Appendix C and answer the following questions.

1.   State the problem of this study.

    a.   Significance: _____

_____

_____

_____

    b.   Background: _____

_____

_____

_____

    c.   Problem statement: _____

_____

_____

_____

2.   State the purpose of this study. _____

_____

Was the purpose clear and concise in this study? **(Yes or No)** Provide a rationale for your answer. _____

_____

_____

_____

3. Are the problem and the purpose significant? **(Yes or No)** Provide a rationale. _____

    _____

    _____

    _____

    _____

    _____

4. Does the purpose identify the concepts and/or variables, population, and setting for this study? _____

    _____

    a. Identify the research concepts and/or variables. _____

        _____

        _____

        _____

    b. Identify the populations. _____

    c. Identify the setting. _____

5. Is it feasible for these researchers to study this problem and purpose? **(Yes or No)** Provide a rationale. _____

    _____

    _____

    _____

    _____

    _____

Objectives, Questions, and Hypotheses

Hallas et al. (2017) Study

Directions: Review this study in Appendix A and answer the following questions.

1. Are objectives, questions, or hypotheses stated in this study? Identify them. _____

    _____

    _____

_____

_____

_____

2. Are they appropriate and clearly stated? **(Yes or No)** Provide a rationale for your answer. _____

_____

_____

_____

_____

Erikson and Davies (2017) Study

Directions: Review this study in Appendix B and answer the following questions.

1. Are objectives, questions, or hypotheses stated in this study? Identify them. _____

_____

2. Are they appropriate and clearly stated? **(Yes or No)** Provide a rationale for your answer. _____

_____

_____

Wendler et al. (2017) Study

Directions: Review this study in Appendix C and answer the following questions.

1. Are objectives, questions, or hypotheses stated in this study? Identify them. _____

_____

_____

_____

_____

2. Are they appropriate and clearly stated for a mixed methods study? **(Yes or No)** Provide a rationale for your answer.

_____

_____

_____

Study Variables or Concepts*

Hallas et al. (2017) Study

Directions: Review this study in Appendix A and answer the following questions.

1. List the major variables in this study and identify the type of each variable (independent, dependent, or research).

Variable	Type of variable

2. Identify the conceptual and operational definitions for the DVD parenting skills intervention.

   a. Conceptual definition: _____

   _____

   _____

   _____

   b. Operational definition: _____

   _____

   _____

3. Are these definitions clear? **(Yes or No)** Provide a rationale for your answer. _____

   _____

   _____

   _____

4. Identify the demographic variables in the study. _____

   _____

   _____

---

*Erikson and Davies (2017) research concepts are discussed in Chapter 3 Introduction to Qualitative Research of this study guide.

Wendler et al. (2017) Study

Directions: Review this study in Appendix C and answer the following questions.

1. List the variables and/or concepts in this study and identify the type of each variable (independent, dependent, or research). Hint: This study focused on description and not on testing the effectiveness of an intervention. The 5- to 10-minute supervised family visit was part of the nurses' care and the study focused on examining the patients' and families' responses to this experience.

Variable or concept	Type of variable or concept

2. Identify the conceptual and operational definitions for the patients' state anxiety.

   a. Conceptual definition of patients' state anxiety: _____

   _____

   _____

   b. Operational definition of patients' state anxiety: _____

   _____

3. Are these definitions clear and concise? **(Yes or No)** Provide a rationale for your answer. _____

    _____

    _____

    _____

    _____

4. Identify the demographic variables in the study. _____

    _____

    _____

Understanding and Critically Appraising the Literature Review

INTRODUCTION

After reading Chapter 6, complete the following exercises. These exercises will assist you in reading and critically appraising research reports and summarizing the findings for use in nursing practice. The answers for the following exercises are in the Answer Key at the back of the book.

EXERCISE 1: TERMS AND DEFINITIONS

Directions: Match each term below with its correct definition. Each term is used only once and all terms are defined.

Terms

a. Article
b. Bibliographic database
c. Citation
d. Clinical journals
e. Conference proceedings
f. Data-based literature
g. Landmark studies
h. Peer reviewed

i. Primary source
j. Reference
k. Relevant studies
l. Replication studies
m. Secondary source
n. Theoretical literature
o. Thesis

Definitions

_____ 1. Source whose author summarizes or quotes content from a primary source.

_____ 2. Periodicals that include research reports and nonresearch articles about professional issues and practice problems.

_____ 3. Reproductions of a study undertaken to determine if the results are the same in different settings or with different samples.

_____ 4. Literature that includes concept analyses, conceptual maps, theories, and conceptual frameworks that support a selected research problem and purpose.

_____ 5. Papers that were evaluated by other scholars as being of high quality, trustworthy, and acceptable for publication.

_____ 6. Source whose author originated or is responsible for generating the ideas published.

_____ 7. Paraphrasing or quoting content from a source, using it as an example, or presenting it as support for a position taken.

_____ 8. A paper about a specific topic published together with similar documents on similar themes in journals, encyclopedias, or edited books.

_____ 9. Research that has a direct bearing on the study being planned or topic of concern.

_____ 10. The author, year, title of a source, and publication information that allows a reader to find the publication to which the author is referring.

_____ 11. Compilations of citations and references that are searchable and allow the researcher to find articles and other publications on a specific topic.

_____ 12. A research project completed by a student as part of the requirements for a master's degree.

_____ 13. Reports of research studies that are published in journals, books, dissertations, and theses.

_____ 14. Compilations of abstracts and papers presented at a professional meeting that may include the findings of pilot studies and preliminary studies.

_____ 15. Significant research projects that influenced a discipline and led to the development of additional studies on the topic.

EXERCISE 2: LINKING IDEAS

Examples of Main Ideas From the Chapter

Directions: Fill in the blanks with the appropriate word(s)/response(s).

1. The process of reviewing the literature has three components, which are (1) finding _____ research reports; (2) _____ _____ the studies; and (3) _____ the study results.

2. The review of the literature identifies what is _____ and what is _____ about a specific topic.

3. A high-quality review of literature contains both _____ and _____ knowledge about a specific topic.

4. Current sources for a literature review are defined as those that were published within _____ years of when the article was accepted for publication.

5. Unlike qualitative studies where the timing and depth of a literature review may vary, the literature review is consistently conducted at the beginning of the research process to direct the planning and implementing of a(n) _____ study.

6. The purpose and timing of the literature review for _____ studies (qualitative approach) is very similar to the purpose and timing of the review for quantitative studies.

7. A well-written summary of a review of the literature provides direction for the formation of the _____ of the study.

8. A(n) _____ is an alphabetized list of topics, each with a compilation of authoritative information on the topic.

9. Although information is readily available online, not all of the information websites provide is
_____, _____, and/or _____.

10. A literature _____ _____ or _____ _____ can be used to help process the information from numerous studies and identify the key aspects of the study (authors, year, purpose, design, sample, measurement methods, and results).

Theoretical and Empirical Sources

Directions: Theoretical and empirical sources are included in the literature review of a published study. Read the sources below and label each with a **T** if it is a theoretical source or an **E** if it is an empirical source. The final determination of the type of source would be made by reviewing the source.

_____ 1. Watson, J. (2008). *Nursing. The philosophy and science of caring* (revised ed.). Boulder, CO: University Press of Colorado.

_____ 2. Abstracts from the Southern Nursing Research Society Conference

_____ 3. Master's thesis

_____ 4. Williams, L. A. (2017). Imogene King's interacting systems theory: Application in emergency and rural nursing. *Online Journal of Rural Nursing and Health Care, 2*(1), 40–50.

_____ 5. Orem, D. E., Taylor, S., & Renpenning, K. M. (2001). *Nursing: Concepts of practice* (6th ed.) St. Louis, MO: Mosby.

_____ 6. Newland, P. K., Lunsford, V., & Flach, A. (2017). The interaction of fatigue, physical activity, and health-related quality of life in adults with multiple sclerosis (MS) and cardiovascular disease (CVD). *Applied Nursing Research, 33*(1), 49–53.

_____ 7. Koehn, A. R., Ebright, P. R., & Draucker, C. B. (2016). Nurses' experiences with errors in nursing. *Nursing Outlook, 64*(6), 566–574.

_____ 8. Doctoral dissertation

_____ 9. von Bertalanffy, L. (1968). *General systems theory.* New York, NY: Braziller.

_____ 10. Moscou-Jackson, G., Allen, J., Kozachik, S., Smith, M. T., Budhathoki, C., & Haywood Jr, C. (2016). Acute pain and depressive symptoms: Independent predictors of insomnia symptoms among adults with sickle cell disease. *Pain Management Nursing, 17*(1), 38–46.

Primary and Secondary Sources

Directions: A literature review includes mainly primary sources. Remember that a primary source is developed by the person conducting the research or developing the theory. A secondary source is the synthesis of primary and other sources. Based on these definitions, determine if a source is primary or secondary. Label each source below with a **P** if it is a primary source or an **S** if it is a secondary source.

_____ 1. Compilation of theories of management

_____ 2. Doctoral dissertation

_____ 3. Theory published by the theorist

_____ 4. Report of a pilot study to test the feasibility of an intervention

_____ 5. Seminal study comparing interventions for stress

_____ 6. Study published in *Applied Nursing Research*

_____ 7. Review of studies to develop an evidence-based practice recommendation

_____ 8. Published review of literature article

_____ 9. Exact replication of a study

_____ 10. Phenomenological research article in *Image: Journal of Nursing Scholarship*

EXERCISE 3: WEB-BASED INFORMATION AND RESOURCES

1. Complete the following questions by finding the specific website to answer the questions.

   a. The National Institute of Nursing Research website is located at:

   _____

   b. On the National Institute of Nursing Research website, the document "Changing Practice, Changing Lives: 10 Landmark Nursing Research Studies" is located at:

   _____

   c. Review the National Institute of Nursing Research document "Changing Practice, Changing Lives: 10 Landmark Nursing Research Studies" to gain a better understanding of landmark studies. Which of the 10 landmark studies do you think is particularly valuable to nursing or your area of interest in nursing? Write the reference for your chosen study in APA format.

   _____

   _____

   _____

2. Use Google Scholar (http://scholar.google.com/) to find the article by Branson, Boss, Padhye, Trötscher, and Ward, published in 2017, about stress in hospitalized children. From the abstract that is available for no charge, answer the following questions.

   a. What is the research design as identified by the researchers?

   _____

   b. What was the sample size? _____

3. Reference management software is a valuable tool to track references obtained through searches. Review information for Endnote located at http://www.endnote.com and RefWorks located at http://www.refworks.com. Based on the information presented on the Endnote and RefWorks websites and any personal experience with the software, which of the two commonly used reference management software would you want to use?

   _____

EXERCISE 4: CONDUCTING CRITICAL APPRAISALS TO BUILD AN EVIDENCE-BASED PRACTICE

Directions: Review the following three articles in Appendices A, B, and C: Hallas, Koslap-Petraco, and Fletcher (2017); Erikson and Davies (2017); and Wendler, Smith, Ellenburg, Gill, Anderson, and Spiegel-Thayer (2017). Use these articles to answer the following questions.

1. The most common way references are cited in nursing publications is APA format (*Publication Manual of the American Psychological Association*, 6th ed., 2010). Knowing the different parts of a reference citation will assist you in locating and recording sources for a formal paper. Please note that APA allows, but does not require, an issue number when a journal has continuous pagination across issues, meaning that the page numbers for Issue 3 begin where the page numbers for Issue 2 end. For example, in *Nursing Research*, the last article in Issue 4 ended on page 335. The first article in Issue 5 started on page 337. In *Understanding Nursing Research*, 7th edition, and this study guide, we have chosen to include issue numbers whenever possible because we have found that knowing the issue number can make finding an electronic article easier. You will notice the reference lists for the study examples may not include an issue number.

   The following source is presented in APA (2010) format as follows:

   > Hallas, D., Koslap-Petraco, M., & Fletcher, J. (2017). Social-emotional development of toddlers: Randomized controlled trial of an office-based intervention. *Journal of Pediatric Nursing, 13*(1), 33–40.

   Please write the category of the citation information in the spaces provided.

   a. In this reference, *Journal of Pediatric Nursing* is the _____.

   b. In this reference, 2017 is the _____.

   c. In this reference, 13 is the _____.

   d. In this reference, 33–40 refers to the _____.

   e. In this reference, 1 represents the _____.

   f. Who is the primary or lead author of this article? _____

   g. What is the title of the article? _____

2. Write the complete reference for the Erikson and Davies (2017) article using APA (2010) format. _____

   _____

   _____

3. Locate the reference list of the Wendler et al. (2017). Several of the references are from the *J PeriAnesth Nurs*, which is the abbreviation for the *Journal of PeriAnesthesia Nursing*.

   a. What is the website for the *Journal of PeriAnesthesia Nursing*?

   _____

   b. Is the *Journal of PeriAnesthesia Nursing* a peer-reviewed journal? (**Yes** or **No**) Provide a rationale for your answer.

   _____

   _____

_____

_____

4. Key words often located near the abstract on the first page of a journal article are helpful tools for future searches on a topic. What key words are listed for the following articles?

   a. Hallas et al. (2017):

   _____

   b. Erikson and Davies (2017):

   _____

   c. Wendler et al. (2017):

   _____

5. The literature review is found in what section(s) of Hallas, Koslap-Petraco, and Fletcher (2017)?

   _____

6. In the review of literature, Erikson and Davies (2017, p. 42) incorporated: "Nurses caring for children at the end of life experience sadness and grief, but offering emotional support to families is an essential aspect of their practice from which they derive meaning and work satisfaction." How many references were used to support this synthesis? _____

Directions: For the next series of questions, critically appraise the review of the literature of the Erikson and Davies (2017) article in Appendix B using the following questions from your _Understanding Nursing Research_, 7th edition, textbook.

7. Quality Sources

   a. Are most references from peer-reviewed sources? (**Yes** or **No**) Provide an example of a peer-reviewed journal on the reference list. _____

   _____

   b. Are most references primary sources? (**Yes** or **No**) Provide an example of one of the primary sources. _____

   _____

   _____

   _____

   _____

   c. Do the authors justify citing references that are not peer-reviewed, primary sources? (**Yes** or **No**) Provide a rationale for your answer. _____

   _____

   _____

d. Did the researchers describe previous studies and relevant theories? (**Yes** or **No**) _____

_____

8. Current Sources

    a. What are the number and percentage of sources published within 10 years and within 5 years of November 20, 2016, when the Erikson and Davies article was accepted for publication? Use the sources provided in the reference list. The percentages will be out of 48 since one of the 49 references has no date ("n.d.").

_____

_____

    b. Are references older than 10 years landmark, seminal, or replication studies? Provide a rationale for your answer.

_____

_____

    c. Are references older than 10 years cited to support measurement methods or theoretical content? Provide support for your answer.

_____

9. Relevant Literature Content

    a. Is the literature content directly related to the study concepts or variables? (**Yes** or **No**) Provide an example.

_____

_____

    b. Are the types of sources and disciplines of the source authors appropriate for the study concepts or variables? (**Yes** or **No**) Provide a rationale for your answer. _____

_____

_____

10. Synthesis of Relevant Content

    a. Are the included studies critically appraised? (**Yes** or **No**) Provide support for your answer.

_____

_____

    b. Are the included studies synthesized? (**Yes** or **No**) Provide support for your answer.

_____

_____

c. Is a clear, concise summary presented of the current empirical and theoretical knowledge in the area of the study, including identifying what is known and not known? (**Yes** or **No**) Provide support for your answer.

_____

_____

_____

_____

d. Does the study address the knowledge gap identified in the literature review? (**Yes** or **No**) Provide support for your answer.

_____

_____

_____

_____

Understanding Theory and Research Frameworks

CHAPTER 7

INTRODUCTION

You need to read Chapter 7 and then complete the following exercises. These exercises will assist you in learning key terms and identifying and critically appraising frameworks in published studies. The answers for the following exercises are in the Answer Key at the back of the book.

EXERCISE 1: TERMS AND DEFINITIONS

Directions: Match each term below with its correct definition. Each term is used only once and all terms are defined.

Terms

a. Abstract
b. Assumptions
c. Concept
d. Concrete
e. Construct
f. Middle range theory
g. Phenomena
h. Philosophies
i. Proposition
j. Research framework
k. Variables

Definitions

_____ 1. An abstract, logical structure of concepts that guides the development of the study and links the study findings to nursing's body of knowledge.

_____ 2. Rational intellectual explorations of truths or principles of being, knowledge, or conduct that influence theory development.

_____ 3. A broader category of ideas that may encompass several concepts.

_____ 4. Statements that are considered true without testing.

_____ 5. A term that abstractly names an object or phenomenon.

_____ 6. A statement that describes the relationships among two or more concepts.

_____ 7. Thinking oriented toward the development of a general idea, without association with a particular instance.

_____ 8. Theories that are less abstract than grand theories; focus on particular patients' health conditions, family situations, and nursing actions; and are often tested in quantitative research.

_____ 9. The conscious awareness of an experience that may be described by a concept, statement, or theory.

_____ 10. Concepts that have been operationally defined so that they can be measured.

_____ 11. Thinking oriented toward a particular instance.

Types of Theories

Directions: Match each type of theory below with its correct definition. Each term is used only once and all terms are defined.

Terms
a. Grand nursing theory
b. Implicit frameworks
c. Practice theory

d. Scientific theory
e. Substantive theory
f. Tentative theory

_____ 1. Middle range theories that are closer to the substance of clinical practice and have clearly identified concepts, definitions of concepts, and relational statements.

_____ 2. Abstract theories that are labeled as conceptual models by some scholars.

_____ 3. Underdeveloped theoretical ideas that may come from the linkages among variables found in other studies that are used to guide a study but are not clearly developed into a research framework.

_____ 4. A newly proposed framework synthesized from the findings of other studies or multiple theories.

_____ 5. Theories of genetics or pathophysiology that are supported by extensive research evidence and whose relational statements may be called *laws*.

_____ 6. Middle range theories that are sometimes called situation-specific theories because they propose interventions for a particular clinical situation.

EXERCISE 2: LINKING IDEAS

Key Theoretical Ideas

Directions: Fill in the blanks with the appropriate word(s)/response(s).

1. The elements of theory are concepts, and statements of the _____ among the concepts.

2. A(n) _____, such as perception of pain, is more specific than a concept and is defined so that it is measurable in a study.

3. The _____ of a theory are tested through research.

4. Statements at the lowest level of abstraction presented in a quantitative study are referred to as _____.

5. How are the conceptual definition and operational definition of a variable different?

_____

_____

_____

6. How are grand nursing theories and middle range theories different? Provide an example of each type of theory.

_____

_____

_____

_____

7. The Self-Care Deficit Theory of Nursing was written by _____.

8. Covell (2008) published a middle range theory of _____

_____.

9. In the study by Reinoso (2016) described in Chapter 7, which middle range theory was used as the framework?

_____

Levels of Abstraction

Directions: Place the following terms in order from the highest to the lowest level of abstraction.

Variable (example – Spiritual Well-being Score)
Construct (example – Holistic Response to Life Stressors)
Operational definition (Participant's total score on the Spiritual Well-being Scale, possible range of 10–50)
Concept (Spiritual Response)

_____ (*highest level of abstraction*)

_____

_____

_____ (*lowest level of abstraction*)

Elements of Theory

Directions: Study the diagram below and answer the following questions in the spaces provided.

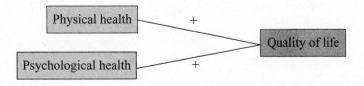

1. List the concepts in the diagram.

    _____

2. What do the arrows represent?

    _____

3. What does this figure represent when included in a study?

    _____

Examples of Frameworks

Directions: Several theories were identified in Chapter 7 that had been used in studies. Match the statement about the theory to the appropriate theorist's name. Hint: Review the middle range theories in Table 7.4 in your textbook, *Understanding Nursing Research*, 7th edition.

Theorist(s)

a. Kolcaba
b. Lenz, Pugh, Milligan, Gift, and Suppe
c. Mishel
d. Meleis
e. Reed
f. Roux, Dingley, and Bush
g. Swanson
h. Thomas

Middle Range Theory

_____   1. The caring aspects of the nurse–patient relationships promote well-being.

_____   2. Comfort is an immediate desirable outcome of nurses' interventions.

_____   3. The middle range theory of women's anger encompasses trait anger as well as modes of anger expression.

_____   4. Nurses are often with persons who are experiencing transitions, changes in their life situations that may affect their health.

_____   5. The interaction of symptoms adds to the complexity of living with illness.

_____   6. Persons facing life-threatening events may acquire an expanded view of self and the environment, a perspective that has been labeled self-transcendence.

_____   7. When facing a new diagnosis, people may experience uncertainty because they do not understand the meaning of the illness-related events and cannot accurately predict the outcome.

_____   8. In managing chronic and terminal illness, women may demonstrate inner strength, a human resource that promotes well-being.

Example of Grand Nursing Theory Used in a Study

Directions: In Chapter 7, find the discussion about the study by Park, Song, and Jeong (2017) and answer the following questions.

1. Describe the sample in the study conducted by Park et al. (2017).

_____

_____

2. Which grand nursing theory was used as the framework for this study?

_____

3. The grand nursing theory was linked to which of the following components of the study? Select one of the answers below.

   a. Design of the study
   b. Development of the intervention
   c. Selection of measurement instruments
   d. Selection of outcome variables

EXERCISE 3: WEB-BASED INFORMATION AND RESOURCES

Directions: Provide the appropriate responses for the following questions in the spaces provided.

1. Kolcaba developed the middle range theory of comfort. Find a web page with information about her theory that includes the three types of comfort that she identified in 1991.

   a. List the three types of comfort identified by Kolcaba:

      1) _____

      2) _____

      3) _____

   b. List the website where you found this information: _____

2. a. Select one of the theories on Table 7.3 and find a website with additional information about the theory. List the website you found here:

   _____

   b. Identify one or two key concepts from the grand theory you selected:

   _____

EXERCISE 4: CONDUCTING CRITICAL APPRAISALS TO BUILD AN EVIDENCE-BASED PRACTICE

Directions: Read and conduct critical appraisals of the framework or theoretical sections of the following research reports.

Hallas, Koslap-Petraco, and Fletcher (2017)

Review the article by Hallas et al. (2017) to answer the first two questions. The article is at the back of the study guide as Appendix A.

1. Which theory did Hallas et al. (2017) identify as the basis for the development of the treatment intervention?

    _____

2. Which specific aspect of the theory did the researchers use to design the treatment intervention?

    _____

3. The following sentence from the Hallas et al. (2017) article describes one of the theoretical statements that supported the study hypotheses.

    "Parental stress has been shown to have a direct negative effect on the psychological health of young children of teenage mothers (Cooper et al., 2009)" (p. 34).

    a. Identify two concepts in the statement. _____

    b. Which hypothesis was based on this theoretical statement? _____

    _____

    _____

    _____

    _____

Wendler, Smith, Ellenburg, Gill, Anderson, and Spiegel-Thayer (2017)

Review the article by Wendler et al. (2017) to answer questions 4–7. The article is at the back of the Study Guide as Appendix C.

4. Which theory was identified as the "theoretical underpinning of the study" (Wendler et al., 2017, p. 47)?

    _____

5. Wendler et al. (2017) linked several aspects of the study to concepts in the theory. Use the list of theoretical concepts to complete the middle column of the following table.
    Concepts from the theory:

    Residual stimuli
    Major contextual stimuli
    Cognitive-emotive and regulator subsystems

    In the last column, find an Internet source that provides a definition for each concept. Write in the concept's definition.

    One helpful site is http://currentnursing.com/nursing_theory/application_Roy's_adaptation_model.html.

    The first concept from the theory and its conceptual definition are identified for you as an example.

Phrases From the Article	Related Concept of the Theory	Conceptual Definition
Overall surgical experience/event	Focal stimuli	The primary threat to adaptation confronting the person right now.
Past healthcare experiences and prior coping for the family as a whole		
Enforcement of separation of patient from family members during phase 1 recovery		
Family visit to mitigate incomplete coping		

6. Which study variable represented the "stress response of both the patient and the family" (Wendler et al. 2017, p. 47)?

   _____

7. Use the critical appraisal questions in Chapter 7 in the *Grove and Gray (2019) Understanding Nursing Research* as an outline for your critical appraisal of the research framework in the Wendler et al. (2017) study.

   _____

   _____

   _____

   _____

   _____

   _____

   _____

   _____

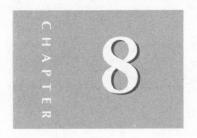

Clarifying Quantitative Research Designs

INTRODUCTION

You need to read Chapter 8 and then complete the following exercises. These exercises will assist you in learning key terms, understanding design validity, and identifying and critically appraising quantitative research designs in published studies. The answers for these exercises are in the Answer Key at the back of the book.

EXERCISE 1: TERMS AND DEFINITIONS

Understanding Common Design Terms

Directions: Match each term below with its correct definition. Each term is used only once and all terms are defined.

Terms

a. Bias
b. Causality
c. Control
d. Correlational design
e. Cross-sectional design
f. Descriptive design
g. Experimental design

h. Longitudinal design
i. Multicausality
j. Noninterventional design
k. Probability
l. Quasi-experimental design
m. Randomized controlled trial (RCT)
n. Research design

Definitions

_____ 1. Blueprint or detailed plan for conducting a study.

_____ 2. Distortion of study findings that are slanted or deviated from the true or expected.

_____ 3. Type of design that facilitates the search for knowledge and examination of causality in situations where control is limited in some ways.

_____ 4. Type of design that involves examining a group of study participants simultaneously in various stages of development, severity of illness, or levels of education to describe changes in a phenomenon across stages.

_____ 5. The power to direct or manipulate factors to achieve a desired outcome. This is greater in experimental than quasi-experimental designs.

_____ 6. Study design that examines relationships between or among two or more variables in a single group.

_____ 7. The recognition that several interrelating variables can be involved in causing a particular outcome.

_____ 8. Descriptive and correlational designs are referred to as these types of designs since the focus is on examining variables as they naturally occur in the environment and not on the implementation of an intervention by researchers.

_____ 9. Research designs conducted to gain information about variables in relatively new areas of study, such as studies to identify problems in current practice, determine trends of illnesses, and categorize information.

_____ 10. Addresses relative rather than absolute causality.

_____ 11. Designs that involve collecting data from the same study participants at different points in time and might also be referred to as repeated measures.

_____ 12. Type of design focused on examining causality where extensive control of the intervention, setting, sampling process, and extraneous variables is possible.

_____ 13. Type of study conducted in nursing and medicine that is noted to be the strongest methodology for testing the effectiveness of an intervention due to the elements of design that limit the potential for bias. These studies are best conducted in multiple geographical locations to increase the sample size and obtain a more representative sample.

_____ 14. Examines the effect of a particular intervention on a selected outcome.

Design Validity Terms

Directions: Match each term below with its correct definition. Each term is used only once and all terms are defined. Review the material in Table 8.1 Types of Design Validity Appraised in Studies in the textbook, _Understanding Nursing Research_, 7th edition, to expand your understanding of design validity.

Terms
a. Construct design validity
b. Design validity
c. Experimenter expectancy
d. External design validity
e. History

f. Internal design validity
g. Low statistical power
h. Mono-operation bias
i. Statistical conclusion design validity
j. Threats to design validity

Definitions

_____ 1. Is a measure of the truth or accuracy of the findings obtained from a study and is focused on overall quality of the study design.

_____ 2. Threat to internal validity that occurs when an event not related to the planned study happens during the study that could have an impact on the findings.

_____ 3. Threat to construct validity where only one measurement method is used to measure a study variable.

_____ 4. Validity focused on determining if study findings are accurate or the result of extraneous variables.

_____ 5. Validity concerned with the fit between the conceptual and operational definitions of the study variables and the quality of the measurement methods used in the study.

_____   6. Validity concerned with whether the conclusions about relationships or differences drawn from statistical analysis are an accurate reflection of the real world.

_____   7. Threat to construct validity where researchers' predictions might bias or influence the outcomes of a study.

_____   8. Problems that exist in a study design and need to be identified in critically appraising a study.

_____   9. Threat to statistical conclusion validity that involves concluding there is no difference between samples when one exists.

_____   10. Validity concerned with the extent to which study findings can be generalized beyond the sample used in the study.

EXERCISE 2: LINKING IDEAS

Directions: Fill in the blanks in this section with the appropriate word(s).

1. According to causality theory, things have causes and causes lead to _____.

2. Quasi-experimental study involves the manipulation of the _____.

3. Quasi-experimental and experimental studies are designed to examine _____

_____.

4. The purpose of quasi-experimental and experimental research designs is to maximize _____ of factors, such as extraneous variables, in the study situation.

5. Coleman (2017, p. 138) conducted a study to examine the association between "health related quality of life and depressive symptoms among seropositive African Americans." This study can be found in the Research Article Library on the Evolve website for *Understanding Nursing Research*, 7th edition, at http://evolve.elsevier. com/grove/understanding. What type of design was used in this study? _____
_____

6. From the perspective of probability theory, a(n) _____ may not produce a specific _____ each time that particular _____ occurs.

7. Critical appraisal of research involves being able to think through threats to _____ that occurred and make judgments about how seriously they affected the integrity of the study findings.

8. Hypothesis: Family history of cardiovascular disease (CVD), smoking, obesity, lack of exercise, and hypertension increase the likelihood of a myocardial infarction in adults. This hypothesis should be tested using a _____ design.

9. In an experimental study, the study participants are randomly assigned to the _____ group or the _____ group.

10. Developing a quality intervention and implementing it consistently in a study using a protocol promotes _____ in the study.

11. A researcher wants to add _____ to the design of a study by limiting the sample to only first-time elderly (>40 years) mothers.

12. The _____ design is used to examine descriptively the differences between two groups, such as the difference between males and females for surgical anxiety.

13. Middle range theories, such as Selye's theory of stress and adaptation and Beck's theory of depression, are usually tested with _____ designs.

14. List three elements of quasi-experimental and experimental designs that are focused on examining causality.

    a. _____

    b. _____

    c. _____

15. Do randomized controlled trials (RCTs) usually have large samples ($N \geq 100$) or small samples ($N \leq 50$)? _____

Determining Types of Design Validity in Studies

Directions: Match the type of design validity with the examples provided from studies. The types of design validity might be used more than once.

Types of Design Validity

a. Construct validity
b. Internal validity
c. External validity
d. Statistical conclusion validity

Study Examples

_____ 1. Over 40% of the potential study participants approached declined to participate because they did not want to follow a structured low-calorie diet. This interaction of the selection of participants and the study intervention is an example of what type of threat to design validity?

_____ 2. A study had a large sample size and statistically significant relationships were found among the variables body mass index (BMI), cholesterol values, and hemoglobin Alc, which indicate what type of design validity?

_____ 3. The Beck Depression Inventory is a valid measure of depression in research, which strengthens what type of design validity?

_____ 4. The study participants were allowed to select either the exercise (intervention) group or the no exercise (comparison) group in a study examining the effects of exercise on weight, BMI, and blood pressure values, which is a threat to what type of design validity?

_____ 5. Researchers and data collectors were blinded to the group receiving the diet educational intervention through a mobile application to strengthen this type of design validity.

_____ 6. An interventional study was conducted in three hospital settings that all had Magnet status and were supportive of research, which strengthens what type of design validity?

_____ 7. Only 10% of the study participants withdrew from a study because of the time constraints and personal and family illnesses, which strengthens which type of design validity?

_____ 8. A diabetic educational program was developed with accuracy and consistently implemented with a protocol in a study, which strengthens what type of design validity?

_____   9. Pain was measured with the Pain Perception Scale and FACES rating scale to strengthen which type of design validity?

_____   10. The study participants were pretested and post-tested to determine a change in their nutrition knowledge following a nutritional educational program. However, the participants noted they could remember the answers to several questions because of the pretest, which is a threat to what type of design validity?

Identifying a Design Model

Directions: Develop models of the appropriate designs in the spaces provided below. Refer to your textbook, *Understanding Nursing Research*, 7th edition, to help you with the different types of designs.

1. Descriptive correlational design:

2. Quasi-experimental pretest and post-test design with a comparison group:

Control and Designs for Nursing Studies

Directions: For each of the questions below, identify the **most** appropriate research design or study and provide a rationale for your answers. What elements might be controlled, if any? Each type of design or study is used only once.

Choices

Comparative descriptive design   Quasi-experimental post-test-only design with comparison group
Correlational study   Quasi-experimental pretest and post-test design with comparison group
Predictive correlational design   Randomized controlled trial (RCT)

1. A study examined the effect on acute pain of showing a DVD of an animated program during the insertion of an IV in children 5 to 7 years of age. The study had intervention and comparison groups and a sample size of 80, with 40 children in each group. The study participants were obtained by a sample of convenience, with 40 children from one hospital unit and 40 children from another unit. The children's acute pain scores were measured with the FACES pain rating scale immediately following the completion of the DVD and IV insertion.

   _____

   _____

   _____

   _____

   _____

2. A sample of 100 first-time mothers was studied to examine the relationships among the variables of hours of sleep, stress level, anxiety level, and depression 1 month after the birth of their infants.

   _____

   _____

   _____

   _____

3. The study included a convenience sample of 80 women with lung cancer who were identified in three oncology centers. The sample size was determined using power analysis. The women's perceived self-esteem, depression level, age, and educational level were used to predict their self-care levels. These variables were measured 3 months into the women's cancer treatments.

   _____

   _____

   _____

   _____

4. A study was conducted to describe and examine differences in health promotion behaviors for males and females with type 2 diabetes. The sample included 100 study participants—50 females and 50 males—that were obtained by a sample of convenience from two primary care clinics.

   _____

   _____

   _____

   _____

5. A study was conducted to examine the effect of vitamins on weight gain in a sample of infants diagnosed with failure to thrive at 2 months after their birth. The sample of 60 infants was obtained from three pediatricians' offices; 30 infants were randomly assigned to the intervention group and 30 to the comparison group. The infants were weighed before and after the implementation of the vitamin intervention, which lasted for 6 months. The intervention was implemented using a structured protocol.

    _____

    _____

    _____

    _____

    _____

6. A study was conducted to examine the effectiveness of a new drug to treat hypertension in adults. The study had a large sample of convenience and included all patients with hypertension in five primary-care clinics in two different cities in Texas. The participants were randomly assigned to either the intervention group or comparison group. The drug intervention was highly controlled to ensure accurate delivery of the medication, and blood pressures (BPs) were precisely measured at the start of the study and 3 months later.

    _____

    _____

    _____

    _____

    _____

EXERCISE 3: WEB-BASED INFORMATION AND RESOURCES

Directions: Answer the following questions with the appropriate website or relevant information.

1. Nurse researchers should follow what guideline for developing, conducting, and reporting a RCT? _____

    _____

    Identify the website for these guidelines: _____

2. Sethares and Asselin (2017, p. 192) conducted a study to examine the "effect of guided reflection on heart failure self-care maintenance and management." Review this study in the Research Article Library on the Evolve website for _Understanding Nursing Research_, 7th edition, at http://evolve.elsevier.com/grove/understanding/, and answer the following questions.

    a. What type of design was used in this study?

        _____

    b. What instrument was used to measure self-care?

        _____

EXERCISE 4: CONDUCTING CRITICAL APPRAISALS TO BUILD AN EVIDENCE-BASED PRACTICE

Hallas, Koslap-Petraco, and Fletcher (2017) Study

Directions: Examine the design of the Hallas et al. (2017) study in Appendix A, and answer the following critical appraisal questions about the design.

1. Identify the type of design conducted in this study. _____

   _____

2. Was the design clearly identified in the research report? (**Yes** or **No**) Provide a rationale for your answer.

   _____

   _____

3. Was an intervention implemented in this study? If so, identify the intervention. _____

   _____

4. Did the design include a comparison or a control group? (**Yes** or **No**) Provide a rationale for your answer.

   _____

   _____

   _____

5. Identify four design validity strengths in the Hallas et al. (2017) study.

   a. _____

   _____

   b. _____

   _____

   c. _____

   _____

   d. _____

   _____

6. Identify two threats to design validity in the Hallas et al. (2017) study.

   a. _____

   _____

b. _____

_____

7. List three methods of control used in the Hallas et al. (2017) study design.

a. _____

b. _____

c. _____

Wendler, Smith, Ellenburg, Gill, Anderson, and Spiegel-Thayer (2017) Study

Directions: Examine the design of the Wendler et al. (2017) study in Appendix C, and answer the following critical appraisal questions about the design.

1. Identify the type of design conducted in the Wendler et al. (2017) study. _____

_____

2. Was the design clearly identified? (**Yes** or **No**) Provide a rationale for your answer. _____

_____

3. Describe the focus of the quantitative part of the Wendler et al. (2017) study design.

_____

_____

_____

_____

4. Identify three design validity strengths in the Wendler et al. (2017) study.

a. _____

_____

b. _____

_____

c. _____

_____

5. Identify two threats to design validity in the Wendler et al. (2017) study.

   a. _____

   _____

   b. _____

   _____

6. Was controlling extraneous variables an important part of this study? (**Yes** or **No**) Provide a rationale for your answer.

   _____

   _____

   _____

Examining Populations and Samples in Research

INTRODUCTION

You need to read Chapter 9 and then complete the following exercises. These exercises will assist you in understanding and critically appraising the sampling process in published studies. The answers to these exercises are in the Answer Key at the back of the book.

EXERCISE 1: TERMS AND DEFINITIONS

Directions: Match each term below with its correct definition. Each term is used only once and all terms are defined.

Terms

a. Accessible population
b. Cluster sampling
c. Convenience sampling
d. Network sampling
e. Nonprobability sampling
f. Probability sampling
g. Purposeful or purposive sampling
h. Quota sampling

i. Simple random sampling
j. Sampling
k. Sampling or eligibility criteria
l. Stratified random sampling
m. Systematic sampling
n. Target population
o. Theoretical sampling

Definitions

_____ 1. Process of selecting a group of people, events, behaviors, or other elements that are representative of the population being studied.

_____ 2. Portion of the target population that the researcher can reasonably contact.

_____ 3. All elements (individuals, objects, events, or substances) that meet the sampling criteria for inclusion in a study.

_____ 4. Judgmental sampling that involves the conscious selection by the researcher of certain participants to include in a study.

_____ 5. List of the characteristics essential for membership in the target population.

_____ 6. Random sampling occurs when every member (element) of the population has a probability higher than zero of being selected for the sample; examples of random sampling methods include simple random sampling, stratified random sampling, cluster sampling, and systematic sampling.

_____ 7. Sampling method that involves selecting every *k*th individual from an ordered list of all members of a population, using a randomly selected starting point.

_____ 8. Most basic random sampling method that involves selection of subjects from the sampling frame for a study.

_____ 9. Random sampling method used when the researcher knows some of the variables in the population that are critical to achieving representativeness; the sample is divided into strata or groups using these identified variables.

_____ 10. Random sampling method in which the sampling frame includes a list of all states, cities, institutions, or organizations that could be in a study; a randomized sample of locations is drawn from this list and subjects are obtained from the selected locations.

_____ 11. Snowballing technique that takes advantage of social groups and the fact that friends tend to hold characteristics in common; participants meeting sample criteria are asked to assist in locating others with similar characteristics.

_____ 12. Nonrandom sampling in which not every element of the population has an opportunity for selection, such as convenience sampling, quota sampling, purposive sampling, network sampling, and theoretical sampling.

_____ 13. Convenience sampling method with an added strategy to ensure the inclusion of study participants who are likely to be underrepresented in the convenience sample, such as women and minority groups.

_____ 14. Sampling method that involves including subjects in a study because they happened to be in the right place at the right time.

_____ 15. A sampling method often used in grounded theory research to develop a selected theory through the research process.

EXERCISE 2: LINKING IDEAS

Directions: Fill in the blanks with the appropriate word(s)/response(s).

1. The individual units of a population are called _____.

2. The sample is obtained from the accessible population and is generalized to the _____
_____ if possible.

3. Representativeness means that the _____, _____
_____, and _____
_____ are alike in as many ways as possible.

4. Identify two ways you might evaluate the representativeness of a sample in a published study.

   a. _____

   b. _____

5. Random variation is _____

   _____.

6. A list of every member of a population is referred to as a(n) _____ _____.

7. A sampling plan outlines the _____.

8. In critically appraising the sampling plan in a quantitative study, what three things might you examine?

   a. _____

   b. _____

   c. _____

9. When the sampling criteria are narrowly defined or very specific, the sample desired is more _____
   _____.

10. When the sampling criteria are broadly defined to include a variety of participants as in a random controlled trial (RCT), the sample desired is more _____.

11. Study participants must be over the age of 18, able to read and write English, newly diagnosed with cancer, and have no other chronic illnesses. These are examples of _____.

12. The sample was 65% female and 40% African American, 30% Hispanic, and 30% Caucasian, which are examples of _____.

13. When nine participants were lost to a study due to complications ($n = 4$), hospitalizations ($n = 3$), and diagnosis of additional illnesses ($n = 2$), this is an example of _____.

14. Identify four types of probability or random sampling.

   a. _____

   b. _____

   c. _____

   d. _____

15. Identify three types of nonprobability or nonrandom sampling commonly used in qualitative research.

   a. _____

   b. _____

   c. _____

16. Have the majority of published nursing studies to date used (**probability [random]** or **nonprobability [nonrandom]**) sampling methods? *(Circle the correct answer.)*

17. The adequacy of the sample size in quantitative studies can be determined by using _____
   _____.

18. Power is the capacity to detect _____ or _____ that actually exist in the population.

19. The minimal acceptable level of power for a study is _____.

20. Effect size is a specific numerical value used to represent the extent to which the _____
   _____ is false.

21. Identify three factors that influence the adequacy of a study's sample size in quantitative studies.

    a. _____

    b. _____

    c. _____

22. Identify three factors that influence the adequacy of a study's sample size in qualitative studies.

    a. _____

    b. _____

    c. _____

23. The two types of sampling criteria that might be included in a study are _____
    and _____ criteria.

24. Calculate the refusal rate for a study in which 250 potential subjects were approached and 208 accepted participation in the study. What percentage of the potential subjects refused to participate?

    _____

25. Calculate the attrition rate for a study with a sample size of 150 and 20 participants withdrew from the study (10 due to increased morbidity, 5 due to time constraints, 3 due to transportation problems, and 2 due to mortality). What was the attrition rate for this study? _____

Sampling Methods for Quantitative and Qualitative Studies

Directions: Match the appropriate sampling method with the example sampling information from a study. Some answer choices are used more than once.

Sampling Method
a. Cluster sampling
b. Convenience sampling
c. Network sampling
d. Purposive sampling
e. Quota sampling

f. Simple random sampling
g. Stratified random sampling
h. Systematic sampling
i. Theoretical sampling

Examples

_____ 1. A sample of 500 nurses was randomly selected from a list of all registered nurses in the state of Texas.

_____ 2. A sample of 50 diabetic patients was obtained from an outpatient clinic then randomly placed in the comparison and intervention groups.

_____ 3. A sample of 10 participants with human immunodeficiency virus (HIV) was obtained by asking three individuals to identify friends with HIV who might participate in the study.

_____ 4. A sample of 1000 critical care nurses was obtained by asking 100 critical care nurse managers in 50 randomly selected, large hospitals to identify 10 staff nurses to complete a survey.

_____ 5. A sample of 90 participants was asked to participate in a study at an immunization booth in the mall.

_____ 6. Gender was used to stratify a sample of 100 randomly selected subjects.

_____ 7. The researcher obtained a list of all certified nurse practitioners, picked a random starting point, and then selected every 25th individual to participate in the study.

_____ 8. A sample of 120 hypertensive subjects was recruited in a clinic to participate in a study.

_____ 9. An equal number of patients with asthma, emphysema, and chronic bronchitis were recruited from the local Better Breathers Chapter and asked to participate in a study.

_____ 10. The sample included 24 patients; 12 were examples of strong self-care and 12 were examples of poor self-care.

_____ 11. A sample of 3000 military personnel was randomly selected to participate in a study.

_____ 12. A sample of 18 drug-addicted nurses was obtained by asking seven participants to identify friends who were drug addicted.

_____ 13. A sample of 17 home health patients was asked to participate in a study because they had what were determined to be stage IV pressure ulcers that were not healing.

_____ 14. A sample of 150 adolescents was obtained at three fast-food restaurants.

_____ 15. A sample of 110 surgery patients was randomly selected from a hospital and randomly placed in control and intervention groups.

_____ 16. Starting from a random point, every 10th subject who entered the emergency department was selected for participation in the study until a sample of 100 was achieved.

_____ 17. A grounded theory study was conducted to develop a theory about individuals and family members' responses to hurricane disasters.

_____ 18. A sample of 120 heart transplant patients was obtained by asking 15 critical care nurse managers in 15 randomly selected, large urban hospitals to identify eight patients to participate in a study.

_____ 19. A sample of 12 participants who had experienced sexual assault was selected for a study; six of them were considered to be coping well after the assault, and six were considered to be coping very poorly after the assault. Data saturation was achieved with these 12 participants.

_____ 20. A sample of 150 participants receiving care in a university health center was asked to participate in a study.

Determining Sample Size for Quantitative and Qualitative Studies

Directions: Match the type of research, quantitative or qualitative, with the criteria for determining the appropriate sample size for a study.

Type of Research

a. Qualitative research
b. Quantitative research
c. Both qualitative and quantitative research

Criteria

_____ 1. Sample size is adequate when saturation of information is achieved in the study area.

_____ 2. The scope of the study influences the sample size; a broad scope requires more participants than does a study with a narrow scope.

_____ 3. Power analysis can be used to determine the sample size for the study.

_____ 4. The quality and the depth of information obtained from the study participants are used to determine the sample size.

_____ 5. As control in the study increases, the necessary sample size decreases.

_____ 6. The more sensitive the measurement methods used in a study, the fewer the participants who are needed.

_____ 7. The broader the scope of the study with more variables or concepts examined, the larger the sample size that is needed.

_____ 8. The sample size needs to be large enough to prevent a Type II error.

_____ 9. Purposive sampling is a common method used to obtain an adequate sample size.

_____ 10. Simple random sampling is the strongest method of decreasing the potential for bias.

EXERCISE 3: WEB-BASED INFORMATION AND RESOURCES

Directions: Provide answers to the questions in this section.

1. Identify a website that has a power analysis calculator. Review the website to improve your understanding of power and power analysis in research articles. _____

2. Identify the website for the World Health Organization (WHO): _____

3. Locate and review information on the WHO Multicentre Growth Reference Study (MGRS) provided on the WHO website. Provide the website URL here: _____
   _____

4. The WHO MGRS led to the development of:

   _____

   _____.

5. What was the approximate sample size for the WHO MGRS?

   _____

6. What six countries were used as the settings for the WHO MGRS?

   _____

7. The large sample size and multiple global settings of the WHO MGRS increased the _____of the sample.

EXERCISE 4: CONDUCTING CRITICAL APPRAISALS TO BUILD AN EVIDENCE-BASED PRACTICE

Hallas, Koslap-Petraco, and Fletcher (2017) Study

Directions: Review the Hallas et al. (2017) study in Appendix A to answer the following questions.

1. Identify the study population. _____

2. List the inclusion sampling criteria and exclusion sampling criteria for this study. Were the sampling criteria clearly stated?_____

   _____

   _____

   _____

   _____

3. Identify the sample characteristics for this study. Is the sample representative of the target population? **(Yes** or **No)** Provide a rationale.

   _____

   _____

   _____

   _____

   _____

4. What is the sample size? Refer to the abstract on page 33 or Table 5 on page 38. _____

5. Was the sample size adequate? Provide a rationale that includes power analysis if it was conducted to determine the necessary sample size. _____

   _____

   _____

   _____

   _____

6. Using data from the abstract on page 33 or Table 5 on page 38, calculate the sample attrition rate for this study.

   _____

   _____

   _____

   _____

   _____

7. Was probability or nonprobability sampling used in this study? _____

8. What specific type of sampling method was used in this study? _____

9. Can the findings be generalized to the target population? Provide a rationale. _____

_____

10. What was the setting for this study? Were the settings natural, partially controlled, or highly controlled?

_____

_____

Erikson and Davies (2017) Study

Directions: Review the Erikson & Davies (2017) study in Appendix B to answer the following questions.

1. Identify the study population. _____

2. List the inclusion and exclusion sampling criteria for this study. _____

_____

_____

_____

_____

3. Identify the sample characteristics for this study. _____

_____

_____

_____

_____

_____

4. What was the sample size? _____

5. Was the sample size adequate? Provide a rationale. _____

_____

_____

_____

6. Was probability or nonprobability sampling used in this study? _____

7. What specific types of sampling methods were used in this study? _____

_____

_____

_____

8. Can the findings be generalized? Provide a rationale. _____

_____

_____

_____

_____

_____

9. What was the setting for this study? Was this setting appropriate? _____

_____

_____

_____

_____

Wendler, Smith, Ellenburg, Gill, Anderson, and Spiegel-Thayer (2017) Study

Directions: Review the Wendler et al. (2017) study in Appendix C and answer the following questions.

1. Identify the study population. _____

_____

2. List the inclusion and exclusion sampling criteria for this study. _____

_____

_____

_____

_____

_____

_____

3. Identify the sample characteristics for this study. Was the sample representative of the target population? (**Yes** or **No**) Provide a rationale.

    _____

    _____

    _____

    _____

    _____

    _____

    _____

4. What was the sample size? _____

5. Was the sample size adequate? Provide a rationale. _____

    _____

    _____

    _____

    _____

6. What was the sample attrition for this study? _____

7. Was probability or nonprobability sampling used in this study? _____

8. What specific type of sampling method was used in this study? _____

9. Can the findings be generalized? Provide a rationale. _____

    _____

    _____

    _____

10. What was the setting for the study? Was the setting natural, partially controlled, or highly controlled? Provide a rationale.

    _____

    _____

    _____

    _____

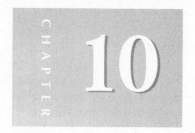

Clarifying Measurement and Data Collection in Quantitative Research

CHAPTER 10

INTRODUCTION

You need to read Chapter 10 and then complete the following exercises. These exercises will assist you in learning key terms and identifying and critically appraising measurement and data collection procedures in published studies. The answers for these exercises are in the Answer Key at the back of the book.

EXERCISE 1: TERMS AND DEFINITIONS

Measurement Concepts and Methods

Directions: Match each term below with its correct definition. Each term is used only once and all terms are defined.

Terms

a. Direct measures
b. Indirect measures
c. Interval-level measurement
d. Interview
e. Likert scale
f. Measurement error
g. Nominal-level measurement
h. Ordinal-level measurement

i. Random measurement error
j. Rating scales
k. Ratio-level measurement
l. Structured observational measurement
m. Systematic measurement error
n. True measure or score
o. Visual analog scale

Definitions

_____ 1. A scale that includes a 100-mm line with anchors on the extreme ends, which might indicate no anxiety before the left anchor and extreme anxiety after the right anchor. Study participants are asked to mark the line where they perceive their anxiety level to be.

_____ 2. Lowest level of measurement when data can be organized into categories that are exclusive and exhaustive, but the categories cannot be rank-ordered.

_____ 3. Error that is the difference between the measurement and true value of a variable that is without a pattern.

_____ 4. A multiple-item scale used to measure perceptions of a phenomenon in a study, such as a 20-item scale used to measure perception of depression with ratings of 1—strongly disagree, 2—disagree, 3—agree, and 4—strongly agree.

_____ 5. Level of measurement with categories that can be rank-ordered, such as levels of functional status—poor functional status, average functional status, and good functional status.

_____ 6. Scaling technique requiring patients to judge the level of their symptoms, such as a nurse asking patients to identify their level of pain on a scale of 1 to 10.

_____ 7. Error that occurs consistently in one direction, such as a scale that weighs everyone 2 pounds less than their true weight, that can alter study results, and must be minimized.

_____ 8. Level of measurement with equal numerical distances between the intervals and an absolute zero point.

_____ 9. Questions posed orally to a study participant as a way of collecting data.

_____ 10. Level of measurement with equal intervals, but without an absolute zero.

_____ 11. Concrete variables (e.g., blood pressure, pulse, and weight) involve these types of measures.

_____ 12. Ideal or perfect measure that does not include error.

_____ 13. Difference between the true measure and the actual measure.

_____ 14. Measurement of abstract ideas (e.g., anxiety, depression, and self-efficacy) involves these types of measures, which are also referred to as indicators.

_____ 15. Measurement method that requires observation of specific elements in a situation.

Reliability, Validity, Accuracy, and Precision in Measurement

Directions: Match each term below with its correct definition. Each term is used only once and all terms are defined.

Terms
a. Accuracy
b. Alternate forms reliability
c. Content validity
d. Evidence of validity from contrasting groups
e. Evidence of validity from convergence
f. Evidence of validity from divergence
g. Internal consistency reliability

h. Interrater reliability
i. Precision
j. Predictive reliability
k. Readability level
l. Reliability
m. Test–retest reliability
n. Validity

Definitions

_____ 1. Determination of how well an instrument or scale reflects the abstract concept being examined.

_____ 2. Addresses the extent to which the physiological instrument or equipment measures what it is supposed to in a study and is comparable to validity for scales.

_____ 3. Concerned with the consistency of a measurement method.

_____ 4. Type of validity where two scales measuring the sample concept like depression are administered to a group at the same time and the study participants' scores on the scales should be positively correlated.

_____ 5. Repeated measures with a scale or instrument to determine the consistency or stability of the instrument in measuring a concept.

_____ 6. Reliability testing used primarily with multi-item scales where each item on the scale is correlated with all of the other items to determine the consistency of the scale in measuring a concept.

_____ 7. Type of validity where an instrument or scale is given to two groups that are expected to have opposite scores, where one group scores high on the scale and another scores low.

_____ 8. Comparison of two observers or judges in a study to determine their equivalence in making observations or judging events.

_____ 9. Examines the extent to which a measurement method includes all of the major elements relevant to the concept being measured; review of scales by experts adds to this type of validity.

_____ 10. Degree of consistency or reproducibility of the measurements made with physiological instruments or equipment; comparable to reliability for scales.

_____ 11. Type of validity where two scales that measure opposite concepts, such as hope and hopelessness, administered to study participants at the same time should result in negatively correlated scores on the scales.

_____ 12. Conducted to determine the study participants' ability to read and comprehend the items on an instrument.

_____ 13. Type of reliability involving a comparison of two paper-and-pencil instruments to determine their equivalence in measuring a concept.

_____ 14. The extent to which an individual's score on a scale or instrument can be used to predict future performance or behavior on a criterion.

Data Collection

Directions: Match each term below with its correct definition. Each term is used only once and all terms are defined.

Terms
a. Administrative data
b. Data collection
c. Data collection plan

d. Primary data
e. Secondary data

Definitions

_____ 1. Detailed plan of how the study will be implemented that is specific to the study being conducted and requires consideration of the common elements of the research process.

_____ 2. Data that are collected for an initial or original study.

_____ 3. The actual process of selecting study participants and gathering data from them during a study.

_____ 4. Data collected for reasons other than research, such as the data collected within clinical agencies.

_____ 5. Data collected during previous research, stored in a database, and later used in other studies to address research questions.

EXERCISE 2: LINKING IDEAS

Directions: Fill in the blanks in this section with the appropriate word(s)/response(s).

1. A fasting blood sugar is an example of what level of measure? _____

2. A reliability value of at least _____ is usually considered a strong coefficient for a scale that has documented reliability and has been used in previous studies.

3. A patient has stage 4 breast cancer. What is the level of measurement for this demographic variable?

   _____

4. Ordinal data have _____ intervals, whereas interval data have _____ intervals.

5. A questionnaire is defined as _____

   _____.

6. The common analysis conducted to determine homogeneity reliability of a scale that has measurement at least at the interval level is the _____.

7. A newly developed multi-item Likert scale to measure hope was administered to a group of patients with depression and had a Cronbach alpha of 0.70. Was the scale (**reliable** or **unreliable**) in this study? *(Circle the correct answer.)* Provide a rationale for your answer: _____

   _____

8. If a study's measurement is not reliable, (**it is** or **it is not**) valid. *(Circle the correct answer.)*

9. Temperature is an example of _____ level of measurement.

10. When critically appraising the measurement section of a study, it is most important for you to examine the _____ and _____ of a scale.

11. A(n) _____ interview includes broad questions and is commonly used in qualitative research.

12. A(n) _____ interview is designed with specific questions to be asked by the researcher and is similar to a questionnaire, which are commonly used in quantitative studies.

13. Which has a higher response rate: (**mailed questionnaire** or **personal interview**)? *(Circle the correct answer.)*

14. Criterion-related validity is strengthened when a study participant's score on an instrument can be used to infer his or her performance on another variable or criterion. Identify the two types of criteria-related validity included in this text: _____ and _____.

15. Describe four situations that might result in error in researchers' measurement of study variables.

    a. _____

    b. _____

    c. _____

    d. _____

Measurement Error

Directions: Match the type of measurement error likely to occur with the measurement methods listed below. You may use the types more than once.

Type of Error
a. Random error
b. Systematic error

Measurement Methods

_____ 1. Community income described for a white, middle-class sample.

_____ 2. Scores on drug calculation tests taken in the morning in a classroom.

_____ 3. Average body weight measured at home, before breakfast every Monday.

_____ 4. Blood pressure taken with equipment that consistently measures the blood pressure high.

_____ 5. Severity of cancer at diagnosis in a community, with patients seeking care at a county hospital.

Levels of Measurement

Directions: Match the level of measurement with the variables or measures listed below. You may use the categories more than once.

Levels of Measurement
a. Nominal
b. Ordinal
c. Interval
d. Ratio

Variables

_____ 1. Body temperature

_____ 2. Gender

_____ 3. Research course grade of 85%

_____ 4. Educational level

_____ 5. Diagnosis of type 2 diabetes

_____ 6. Severity of illness level

_____ 7. Score from visual analog scale

_____ 8. Hemoglobin A1c value

_____ 9. Depression score obtained using the Center for Epidemiologic Studies Depression Scale

_____ 10. Registered nurse licensure exam—passed

_____ 11. Length of hospital stay

_____ 12. Type of cancer

_____ 13. Pain score from Wong-Baker FACES Pain Rating Scale

_____ 14. Body mass index (BMI)

_____ 15. Marital status

_____ 16. Years of work experience

_____ 17. Income measured as: <$60,000; $60,000–70,000; >$70,000

_____ 18. Hospital versus rehabilitation care

_____ 19. Ethnicity/race

_____ 20. Systolic and diastolic blood pressure

Scales

Directions: Identify the type of scale being presented in the following examples.

Type of Scale
a. Likert scale
b. Rating scale
c. Visual analog scale

Examples

_____ 1. State-Trait Anxiety Inventory (STAI)

_____ 2. No Pain |——| Most Severe Pain Possible

_____ 3. On a scale of 1 to 10, how anxious are you feeling?

Sensitivity and Specificity

Directions: Answer the questions in this section.

1. Complete the table below on sensitivity and specificity.

Diagnostic Test Results	Disease Present	Disease Absent or Not Present
Positive test	*a* (true positive)	
Negative test		

2. What is the formula for sensitivity?_____

3. What is the formula for specificity?_____

Sensitivity and Specificity of Colonoscopy Screening Tests

Diagnostic Test Results	Disease Present	Disease Absent or Not Present	Totals
Positive test	250	50	300
Negative test	40	750	790
Totals	290	800	1090

4. What is the number of false positives for the colonoscopy screening test in the previous table? _____

5. What is the percentage of false positives for the colonoscopy screening test using the data in the previous table?

_____

6. What is the number of false negatives for the colonoscopy screening test? _____

7. What is the percentage of false negatives for the colonoscopy screening test? _____

8. What is the sensitivity of the colonoscopy screening test? _____

9. What is your interpretation of the sensitivity value? _____

10. What is the specificity of the colonoscopy screening test? _____

11. What is the positive likelihood ratio (LR) formula? _____

12. What is the positive LR for the colonoscopy screening test? _____

13. What is your interpretation of the positive LR value? _____

14. What is the negative LR formula? _____

15. What is the negative LR for the colonoscopy screening test? _____

16. What is your interpretation of the negative LR value? _____

EXERCISE 3: WEB-BASED INFORMATION AND RESOUCES

Directions: Complete the following questions.

1. Search for and identify the Agency for Healthcare Research and Quality (AHRQ) National Quality Measures Guideline website:

   _____

   Review the resources that are available on this website.

2. Search for a national website that discusses the Center for Epidemiologic Studies Depression Scale Revised (CES-R). Identify this website:

   _____

   Review the materials that are available on the CES-R.

3. There is a CES-R scale to screen children for depression. Locate a website that describes this scale:

   _____

4. Identify the website for the Wong-Baker FACES pain rating scale: _____

   _____

5. Wendler et al. (2017) measured stress for patients and family members with the State-Trait Anxiety Inventory (STAI) by Spielberger. Locate a website for this scale and review the relevant information:

   _____

EXERCISE 4: CONDUCTING CRITICAL APPRAISALS TO BUILD AN EVIDENCE-BASED PRACTICE

Directions: Review the quantitative research article in Appendix A and the mixed methods study in Appendix C and answer the following critical appraisal questions in the spaces provided.

Hallas, Koslap-Petraco, and Fletcher (2017) Study

1. Identify the measurement methods for dependent variables in the Hallas et al. (2017) study in the following table. Also indicate whether the instruments are a direct or indirect method of measuring the study variables.

Variables	Measurement Methods	Direct or Indirect Measurement Method
Maternal confidence		
Social-emotional development of toddlers		

2. Describe key reliability and validity information for the measurement methods in the Hallas et al. (2017) study.

Variables	Measurement Methods' Reliability and Validity
Maternal confidence	
Social-emotional development of toddlers	

3. Critically appraise the quality of the measurement of maternal confidence.

_____

_____

_____

_____

_____

_____

4. Critically appraise the quality of the measurement of social-emotional development of toddlers. _____

_____

_____

_____

_____

_____

5. Identify some of the key ideas from the data collection process for the Hallas et al. (2017) study.

_____

_____

_____

_____

_____

_____

_____

6. Critically appraise the quality of the data collection process in the Hallas et al. (2017) study.

_____

_____

_____

_____

Wendler, Smith, Ellenburg, Gill, Anderson, and Spiegel-Thayer (2017) Study

1. Identify the measurement methods for selected variables in the Wendler et al. (2017) study (see Appendix C) in the following table. Indicate whether the scales are a direct or indirect method of measuring the study variables.

Variable(s)	Measurement Method(s)	Direct or Indirect Measurement Method
State anxiety		
Satisfaction with visit		

2. Identify key ideas about the reliability and validity of the following measurement methods from the Wendler et al. (2017) study.

Variables	Scales' Reliability and Validity Information From the Wendler et al. (2017) Study
State anxiety	
Satisfaction with visit	

3. Critically appraise the reliability and validity of the STAI.

_____

_____

_____

_____

_____

4. Critically appraise the reliability and the validity of the "satisfaction with visit scale."

_____

_____

_____

_____

5. Identify the precision and accuracy for the measurement of vital signs in the Wendler et al. (2017) study.

Variables	Measurement Method and Reported Precision and Accuracy in This Study
Vital signs (VSs)—Mean blood pressure and heart rate	

6. Critically appraise the precision and accuracy of measurement of VSs.

   _____

   _____

   _____

7. Describe key ideas from the data collection process for the Wendler et al. (2017) study.

   _____

   _____

   _____

   _____

   _____

   _____

   _____

8. Critically appraise the quality of the data collection process in the Wendler et al. (2017) study. (Hint: Review the flow diagram in Figure 1).

   _____

   _____

   _____

   _____

   _____

   _____

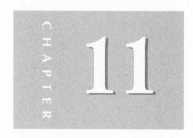

Understanding Statistics in Research

INTRODUCTION

You need to read Chapter 11 and then complete the following exercises. These exercises will assist you in learning key terms and identifying and critically appraising statistical techniques, results, and discussion sections in published studies. The answers to these exercises are in the Answer Key at the back of the book.

EXERCISE 1: TERMS AND DEFINITIONS

Directions: Match each term below with its correct definition. Each term is used only once and all terms are defined.

Terms

a. Alpha
b. Decision theory
c. Descriptive statistics
d. Effect size
e. Generalization
f. Implications for nursing
g. Independent groups
h. Inferential statistics
i. Outliers
j. Paired (dependent) groups
k. Posthoc analysis
l. Power
m. Probability theory
n. Type I error
o. Type II error

Definitions

_____ 1. Findings acquired from a specific study that are applied to a target population.

_____ 2. Summary statistics that allow researchers to organize data in ways that give meaning and facilitate insight.

_____ 3. Error that occurs with the acceptance of the null hypothesis when it is false.

_____ 4. Indicates the "degree to which a phenomenon is present in a population," such as the strength of a relationship between two variables, or "the degree to which the null hypothesis is false."

_____ 5. Level of significance that is set at the start of a study.

_____ 6. Theory used to explain the extent of a relationship, the likelihood an event will occur in a given situation, or the likelihood that an event can be accurately predicted.

_____ 7. Study participants with extreme values that seem unlike the rest of the sample.

_____ 8. Error that occurs with the rejection of the null hypothesis when it is true.

_____ 9. Theory with the assumption that all of the groups used to test a particular hypothesis are components of the same population relative to the variables under study.

_____ 10. The meaning of research findings for the body of nursing knowledge, theory, policy, and practice.

_____ 11. Groups are formed so the selection of one study participant is unrelated to the selection of other participants.

_____ 12. Data analysis after an analysis of variance (ANOVA) to determine differences among three or more groups.

_____ 13. The probability that a statistical test will detect a significant difference or relationship that exists.

_____ 14. Statistics designed to address objectives, questions, or hypotheses in studies to allow extension of findings from the study sample to the target population.

_____ 15. Study participants or observations selected for data collection are related in some way to the selection of other participants or observations.

EXERCISE 2: LINKING IDEAS

Directions: Fill in the blanks with the appropriate word(s)/response(s).

1. The purpose of statistical analysis is to _____

    _____.

2. List three steps that researchers conduct during the data analysis process to determine the results for their study.

    a. _____

    b. _____

    c. _____

3. List three statistical analysis techniques conducted to describe the sample characteristics in a study.

    a. _____

    b. _____

    c. _____

4. List five different types of results obtained from the statistical analyses conducted for quasi-experimental and experimental studies.

    a. _____

    b. _____

    c. _____

    d. _____

    e. _____

5. Identify five major ideas or content areas included in the discussion section of a research report.

a. _____

b. _____

c. _____

d. _____

e. _____

6. Draw and label a normal curve with a mean of 0 and a standard deviation of 1.

7. In a normal distribution of scores, what percent of the scores fall between −1.96 and +1.96 standard deviations of the mean? _____.

8. The most precise level of statistical significance is achieved by conducting a (**one-tailed** or **two-tailed**) level of significance. *(Circle the correct answer.)*

9. A _____ error occurs if you say that a therapeutic touch intervention works to relieve acute pain when it does not.

10. An analysis of variance is conducted on study data to determine (**relationships** or **group differences**). *(Circle the correct answer.)*

11. The measure of central tendency calculated for nominal level data is _____.

12. A measure of dispersion that is calculated for interval and ratio level data is _____.

13. What does "n" represent in a statistical table that includes the results from the intervention and comparison groups in a study? _____

14. A diagram of points placed at the study participants' relative scores along a best fit line is called a(n) _____ _____.

15. Data analysis that is conducted on two variables is called _____.

Linking Statistics With Analysis Techniques

Directions: Match each statistic with its appropriate analysis technique. Each statistic is used only once, and all analysis techniques have a statistic included.

Statistics

a. *df*
b. *SD*
c. *r*
d. *ES*
e. *R*

f. *F*
g. χ^2
h. %
i. *t*
j. α

Analysis Techniques

_____ 1. Alpha

_____ 2. Analysis of variance

_____ 3. Chi-square

_____ 4. Degrees of freedom

_____ 5. Effect size

_____ 6. Pearson product-moment correlation

_____ 7. Percentage

_____ 8. Regression analysis

_____ 9. Standard deviation

_____ 10. *t*-test

Linking Levels of Measurement With Analysis Techniques

Directions: Link the appropriate level of measurement for data to be analyzed by each of the following analysis techniques. The levels of measurement can be used more than once. Some of the statistical analyses can be used for two different levels of measurement. (Hint: Review Figure 11.8, Statistical Decision Tree or Algorithm for Identifying an Appropriate Analysis Technique, in your textbook *Understanding Nursing Research*, 7th ed.)

Levels of Measurement for Data

a. Nominal level
b. Ordinal level
c. Interval/ratio level

Statistical Analysis Techniques

_____ 1. *t*-test for independent groups

_____ 2. Chi-square

_____ 3. Mean

_____ 4. Pearson product-moment correlation

_____ 5. Percentages

_____ 6. Median

_____ 7. Regression analysis

_____ 8. Effect size

_____ 9. Standard deviation

_____ 10. Range

_____ 11. Mode

_____ 12. Ungrouped frequencies

_____ 13. Analysis of variance

_____ 14. *t*-test for paired or dependent groups

_____ 15. Grouped frequencies

Statements, Inferences, and Generalizations

Directions: Match the statement category with its example study. Each statement category is used only once.

Statement Categories
a. Decision theory statement
b. Probability theory statement
c. Inference
d. Generalization

Example Studies

_____ 1. The experimental pain assessment tool can be used to accurately assess pain levels in hospitalized adult patients after many different types of surgery.

_____ 2. This type of statement suggests that when stress occurs, disruption in social activity and mood are likely to occur.

_____ 3. No significant differences were found in functional outcomes between the two groups of patients treated with sterile petroleum gauze or sterile nonmedicated gauze.

_____ 4. Because most major risk factors thought to affect mental health did not change, and no adverse changes in sleepiness were observed during the intervention period, it is plausible to argue that the music intervention would not have reduced insomnia reports over longer time periods.

Describing the Sample

Directions: Referring to the table below, answer the questions that follow in the spaces provided.

Nurses (N = 100)	Frequency (f)	Percentage (%)
Age in Years		
18–29	10	10%
30–39	20	20%
40–49	35	35%
50–59	30	30%
60 and greater	5	5%
Nursing Education		
Associate's Degree in Nursing (ADN)	50	50%
Diploma	20	20%
Bachelors' of Science in Nursing (BSN)	30	30%
Nurses' Years of Experience	Mean(M) = 15.5 (SD = 2.1)	Range = 1 to 35 years

1. Which variable contains grouped data? _____

2. What is the mode of "Nursing Education"? _____

3. Which "Age Group" is the median? _____

4. What is the standard deviation for the "Nurses' Years of Experience"? _____

5. What is the most years of experience that the nurses have in this example? _____

6. Ninety-five percent (95%) of the nurses' years of experience are between what years? Round your answer to two decimal places.

   _____

   _____

Measures of Central Tendency

Directions: Referring to the results of a 10-item Likert scale with response options of 1 to 5, printed below, answer the questions in the spaces provided.

mean = 3.42   SD = 0.76
median = 3.10   mode = 3.00

1. Which value is the average? _____

2. Which value is the 50th percentile? _____

3. What does the mode represent? _____

4. Using the *SD* value, calculate the range of values ±1 *SD* from the mean. _____

   _____

   _____

Name That Statistical Analysis Technique!

Directions: Match the following statistical analysis results with the correct analysis technique. Identify the purpose of each analysis technique and the level of measurement (i.e., nominal, ordinal, interval, or ratio) required for conducting the technique.

Statistical Analysis Results

a. $\chi^2 = 4.61$ $df = 2$ $p = 0.10$
b. $t = 15.631$ $df = 180$ $p = 0.001$
c. $r = -0.315$ $df = 76$ $p < 0.05$
d. $F = 36.71$ $df = 420$ $p < 0.001$

Statistical Analysis Techniques

_____ 1. ANOVA

Purpose of analysis: _____

Level of measurement of data analyzed with this technique: _____

_____ 2. Chi-square

Purpose of analysis: _____

Level of measurement of data analyzed with this technique: _____

_____

_____ 3. Pearson product-moment correlation

Purpose of analysis: _____

Level of measurement of data analyzed with this technique: _____

_____ 4. *t*-test

Purpose of analysis: _____

Level of measurement of data analyzed with this technique: _____

Significance of Results

Directions: In the following statistical findings, indicate whether the results were statistically significant (*) or not statistically significant (NS), assuming a level of significance set at alpha = 0.05. You may use each category more than once.

* = Statistically significant
NS = Not statistically significant

_____ 1. $\chi^2 = 1.61$ $df = 2$ $p = 0.10$

_____ 2. $t = 15.631$ $df = 180$ $p = 0.001$

_____ 3. $r = -0.315$ $df = 76$ $p < 0.05$

_____ 4. $F = 1.37$ $df = 25$ $p = 0.23$

_____ 5. $R = .576$ $df = 130$ $p = <0.001$

EXERCISE 3: WEB-BASED INFORMATION AND RESOURCES

Directions: Answer the following questions with the appropriate website or relevant information.

1. Identify a website that provides a program for calculating power analysis for a study sample size or the power of a study results. _____

2. What does SPSS stand for?

   _____

3. Identify a website that provides introductory information about SPSS:

   _____

   _____

4. The following workbook can provide you additional information about statistical analysis and assist you in critically appraising the results sections of published studies:

   Grove S. K., & Cipher, D. J. (2017). *Statistics for nursing research: A workbook for evidence-based practice* (2nd ed.). St. Louis, MO: Elsevier.

   Locate this resource on the Elsevier website and on an Amazon website:

   _____

   _____

5. Locate the following study in the Research Article Library on the Evolve website for *Understanding Nursing Research*, 7th edition, at http://evolve.elsevier.com/grove/understanding/:

   Coleman, C. L. (2017). Health related quality of life and depressive symptoms among seropositive African Americans. *Applied Nursing Research, 33*(1), 138–141.

   a. What descriptive statistics were conducted to describe the sample in this study? _____

      _____

      _____

   b. What key inferential statistics were conducted in this study? _____

      _____

      _____

   c. What were the purposes of these analysis techniques in the previous question? _____

      _____

      _____

   d. What future studies were recommended by Coleman (2017)? _____

      _____

      _____

EXERCISE 4: CONDUCTING CRITICAL APPRAISALS TO BUILD AN EVIDENCE-BASED PRACTICE

Hallas, Koslap-Petraco, and Fletcher (2017)

Directions: Read the Hallas et al. (2017) study found in Appendix A and then answer the following questions in the spaces provided.

1. How many groups did this study have, and what were the names of the groups? _____

    _____

2. How were the groups developed in the study? _____

3. Were the groups independent or paired (dependent) in this study? _____

4. For each variable in the table, indicate the level of measurement (i.e., nominal, ordinal, interval, or ratio) and the descriptive analysis technique(s) that were conducted in the Hallas et al. (2017) study.

Demographic and Study Variables	Level of Measurement	Descriptive Analysis Techniques
Race/Ethnicity		
Occasional help from babysitter		
Toddler goes to day care		
Other children in the home		
Mother works full or part time		
Mother's age (years)		
Baby's age (months)		
Toddler Care Questionnaire (TCQ) scores at baseline (pretest) and post-test results		
Brigance Toddler Screen scores at baseline (pretest) and post-test results		

5. a. Were the groups' demographic characteristics and pretest baseline scores for the TCQ and Brigance significantly different?

_____

_____

b. Is this a strength or weakness in the Hallas et al. (2017) study?

_____

c. Provide a rationale for your answer:

_____

_____

_____

6. What inferential statistic was conducted to analyze the TCQ and Brigance scores and what was the purpose of this statistic? Hint: See Hallas et al. (2017, p. 39) Tables 7 and 8. _____

_____

_____

7. What were the results for the TCQ pretest and post-test for the treatment and control groups? Was the intervention effective in this study?

_____

_____

_____

_____

8. Identify if hypotheses 1 and 2 were supported or not supported in this study.

_____

_____

9. The following result was found on page 38 of the Hallas et al. (2017) study: $t(57) = 2.079, p = 0.042$

a. Is this result statistically significant? (**Yes** or **No**) Provide a rationale for your answer:

_____

_____

b. Is this result clinically important? (**Yes** or **No**) Provide a rationale for your answer: _____

_____

_____

10. What were the limitations of this study? Do these limitations help explain the study findings?

_____

_____

_____

_____

_____

_____

_____

_____

11. Should these findings be implemented in practice now or is additional research recommended before use? Provide a rationale for your answer: _____

_____

_____

_____

_____

Wendler, Smith, Ellenburg, Gill, Anderson, & Spiegel-Thayer (2017) Study

Directions: Read the Wendler et al. (2017) study found in Appendix C and then answer the following questions in the spaces provided.

1. For each variable in the table, indicate the level of measurement (i.e., nominal, ordinal, interval, or ratio) and the descriptive analysis technique(s) that were conducted in the Wendler et al. (2017) study.

Demographic Variables	Level of Measurement	Descriptive Analysis Techniques
Patient and family member's age (years)		
Patient and family member's race		
Patient and family member's gender		

2. What was the design of this study? _____

3. The study included a single group that had (**independent** or **paired [dependent]**) score. _(Circle the correct answer.)_ Provide a rationale for your answer: _____

_____

4. What inferential statistic was conducted to examine the differences between the pretest and post-test state anxiety scores for the patients and family members? _____

   Was this technique appropriate? (**Yes** or **No**) Provide a rationale for your answer: _____

   _____

   _____

   _____

5. The following result was obtained from Table 2 (p. 52): $t = 5.63$, $p < .001$

   a. Is this result statistically significant? _____

   b. What does this result mean? _____

      _____

      _____

6. a. What analysis techniques were conducted on the mean blood pressure (MBP) and heart rate (HR) physiological responses before and at the end of the visit? _____

   b. Were these statistical techniques appropriate? (**Yes** or **No**) Provide a rationale for your answer: _____

      _____

      _____

7. a. Were the MBP and HR significantly different for the patient after the family visit?

      _____

   b. Provide a rationale for your answer: _____

      _____

      _____

8. Did the researchers generalize their findings? Was this appropriate based on the study findings? _____

   _____

   _____

   _____

   _____

   _____

9. Identify key conclusions from the Wendler et al. (2017) study. Were they appropriate? _____

   _____

   _____

_____

_____ _____

_____

_____

_____

_____

_____

_____

10. How were data collected for the qualitative part of the Wendler et al. (2017) study? _____

_____

_____

11. What were the key qualitative results for the Wendler et al. (2017) study?

_____

_____

_____

_____

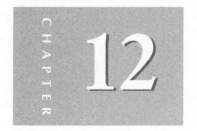

Critical Appraisal of Quantitative and Qualitative Research for Nursing Practice

INTRODUCTION

You need to read Chapter 12 and then complete the following exercises. These exercises will assist you in understanding the quantitative and qualitative research critical appraisal processes. The answers to these exercises are in the Answer Key at the back of the book.

EXERCISE 1: TERMS AND DEFINITIONS

Directions: Match each term below with its correct definition. Each term is used only once and all terms are defined.

Terms
a. Confirmability
b. Critical appraisal
c. Dependability
d. Refereed journals
e. Transferable
f. Credibility

Definitions

_____ 1. Applicability of qualitative findings to other settings with similar participants.

_____ 2. Published collections of articles that have been critically appraised by expert peer reviewers.

_____ 3. Degree of readers' confidence that the findings from a qualitative research report represent the perspectives of the participants.

_____ 4. The documentation of the steps taken and the decisions made during data analysis in a qualitative study.

_____ 5. Examination of the quality of studies to determine the credibility, significance, and meaning of the findings for nursing.

_____ 6. Extent to which other researchers can review the audit trail of a qualitative study and agree that the authors' conclusions are logical.

EXERCISE 2: LINKING IDEAS

Directions: Fill in the blanks with the appropriate word(s).

1. An intellectual research critical appraisal involves careful examination of all aspects of a study to judge the

   _____, _____, _____,

   and _____ of the study.

2. Identify three important questions that are part of an intellectual research critical appraisal.

   a. _____

   b. _____

   c. _____

3. Identify at least three reasons why you would critically appraise nursing studies.

   a. _____

   b. _____

   c. _____

4. Adherence to ethical standards in nursing involves protecting study participants' _____
   and obtaining _____ _____ from the participants.

5. In qualitative research, what components should be included in the abstract?

   a. _____

   b. _____

   c. _____

   d. _____

Determination of Quantitative Study Strengths and Weaknesses

Directions: Read the quantitative examples below and label each with **S** if it is a **strength** of the study or **W** if it is a **weakness** of the study.

Examples

_____ 1. The study framework does not clearly link to the study variables' conceptual definitions.

_____ 2. The principal investigator of the hypertension study is a PhD-prepared RN with 20 years of clinical experience in cardiac care.

_____ 3. The depression scale used in a study of depression and quality of life in multiple sclerosis patients was newly developed by the researcher and had never been used in a study.

_____ 4. Researchers did not describe a protocol for training to ensure consistency among the multiple care providers who implemented the study's counseling intervention.

_____ 5. The research design is linked to the sampling method, study instruments, and statistical analyses.

_____ 6. The findings of this replication study are consistent with the findings of previous studies.

_____ 7. Network sampling was used to recruit participants.

_____ 8. Power analysis conducted prior to data collection showed a need for 25 participants for each of the two groups. A total of 55 participants were recruited with 28 randomized into the intervention group and 27 into the control group.

_____ 9. Researchers reported three significant results without reporting the level of significance (alpha).

_____ 10. An experimental study of a weight loss intervention implemented using a detailed protocol for consistent weighing of study participants on high precision scales wearing pre-weighed hospital gowns.

_____ 11. A power analysis was not conducted prior to the start of the two group experimental study.

_____ 12. The study of handwashing cleansing agents was a double blind randomized controlled trial.

_____ 13. Stratified random sampling was used to recruit participants.

_____ 14. Of the 25 references cited in a quasi-experimental study focused on a weight loss program, 5 (20%) were published within the 5 years of article acceptance and 10 (40%) were published within the 10 years of article acceptance.

_____ 15. Prior to data collection, the institutional review board (IRB) from the researcher's university granted approval for a study of directly observed therapy of tuberculosis in homeless individuals.

Determination of Qualitative Study Strengths and Weaknesses

Directions: Read the qualitative examples below and label each with **S** if it is a **strength** of the study or **W** if it is a **weakness** of the study.

Examples

_____ 1. All of the references cited in the ethnographic research article were from peer-reviewed journals except for a book on ethnography.

_____ 2. Researchers label the study as qualitative but don't identify the specific qualitative approach used.

_____ 3. The review of literature did not justify the study purpose because a gap in nursing knowledge was not identified.

_____ 4. Study interviews were audio recorded and then typed word for word to create a verbatim narrative.

_____ 5. In a study of the lived experience of domestic violence, the researcher described the study protocol if participants became upset during the study interview, which included cessation of the interview and referral to community resources.

_____ 6. Several data inconsistencies and grammatical errors are noted in the ethnographic study article.

_____ 7. Prior to data collection, for a study on the lived experience of frequent loss among pediatric hospice nurses, the researcher obtained informed consent and participants signed written consent forms.

_____ 8. The grounded theory study was conducted by two RNs with bachelor's degrees in nursing.

_____ 9. The in-depth interviews and detailed observations provided rich data.

_____ 10. Evidence of an audit trail was included in the research report.

_____ 11. The abstract of a grounded theory study included the study's purpose, grounded theory as the specific qualitative methodology, sample, and key results.

_____ 12. The study's sample exclusion criteria were the opposite of the sample inclusion criteria.

_____ 13. The study findings were linked to specific quotes or observations.

_____ 14. Interviews for a phenomenology study were conducted at a busy nurses' station at a university hospital.

_____ 15. The sample size of 18 participants was determined by data saturation.

EXERCISE 3: WEB-BASED INFORMATION AND RESOURCES

Directions: Search, locate, and review the websites identified in the following questions.

1. The Quality and Safety Education for Nurses (QSEN) Project has defined quality and safety competencies for nursing and proposed the knowledge, skills, and attitudes (KSAs) to be developed in nursing prelicensure programs for each competency. These KSAs are for students in baccalaureate programs who are seeking to become registered nurses (RNs). Locate the QSEN website for the pre-licensure KSAs:

   _____

2. Identify the six QSEN competency areas for pre-licensure nursing students:

   a. _____

   b. _____

   c. _____

   d. _____

   e. _____

   f. _____

3. Which QSEN competency is the most closely linked to understanding the research process and critically appraising studies?

   _____

4. Which evidence-based practice (EBP) attitude is focused on critical appraisal of studies?

   _____

5. Which EBP skill is focused on reading, understanding, and evaluating studies?

   _____

6. The Magnet Recognition Program was developed by the American Nurses Credentialing Center (ANCC) to recognize healthcare agencies for quality patient care, nursing excellence, and innovations in professional nursing, which requires reading, critically appraising, and applying relevant research knowledge in practice. Identify the Magnet Recognition Program website:

_____

7. Search for and identify the website that lists the clinical agencies that have Magnet status:

_____

Review the agencies on this website. Whether an agency has Magnet status is important when evaluating potential employers.

EXERCISE 4: CONDUCTING CRITICAL APPRAISALS TO BUILD AN EVIDENCE-BASED PRACTICE

Directions: Read the research articles in Appendices A and B. Conduct a critical appraisal using the guidelines provided in Boxes 12.2 and 12.3 in your textbook, *Understanding Nursing Research*, 7th edition.

1. Conduct a critical appraisal of the Hallas, Koslap-Petraco, and Fletcher (2017) article using the **quantitative** guidelines outlined in **Box 12.2** in your textbook. Many parts of this study were critically appraised in the earlier chapters of this study guide.

   a. Writing quality

   _____

   b. Title

   _____

   c. Authors

   _____

   d. Abstract

   _____

   e. Research problem

   _____

   f. Purpose

   _____

   g. Literature review

   _____

   h. Framework or theoretical perspective

   _____

   i. Research objectives, questions, or hypotheses

   _____

j. Variables

_____

k. Research design

_____

l. Sample

_____

m. Setting

_____

n. Measurement

_____

o. Data collection

_____

p. Data analyses

_____

q. Interpretation of findings

_____

r. Limitations

_____

s. Conclusions

_____

t. Nursing implications

_____

u. Future research

_____

v. Critique summary

_____

2. Conduct a critical appraisal of the Erikson and Davies (2017) article using the **qualitative** guidelines outlined in **Box 12.3** of your textbook, *Understanding Nursing Research*, 7th edition. Many parts of this study were critically appraised earlier in this study guide (see Chapter 3 focused on qualitative research).

a. Writing quality

_____

b. Title

_____

c. Authors

_____

d. Abstract

_____

e. Research problem

_____

f. Purpose

_____

g. Literature review

_____

h. Study framework or philosophical orientation

_____

i. Research objectives (aims) or questions

_____

j. Qualitative approach

_____

k. Sample

_____

l. Setting

_____

m. Data collection

_____

n. Data analysis

_____

o. Interpretation of findings

_____

p. Limitations

_____

q. Conclusions

_____

r. Nursing Implications

_____

s. Future research

_____

t. Critique summary

_____

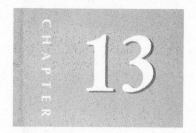

Building an Evidence-Based Nursing Practice

INTRODUCTION

You need to read Chapter 13 and then complete the following exercises. These exercises will assist you in reading and critically appraising research syntheses commonly published in nursing, including systematic reviews, meta-analyses, meta-syntheses, and mixed methods systematic reviews. Exercises are also provided to assist you in implementing research evidence in your practice. The answers to these exercises are in the Answer Key at the back of the book.

EXERCISE 1: TERMS AND DEFINITIONS

Directions: Match each term with its correct definition. Each term is used only once and all terms are defined.

Terms

  a. Algorithms
  b. Best research evidence
  c. Evidence-based practice (EBP)
  d. Evidence-based practice centers (EPCs)
  e. Evidence-based practice guidelines
  f. Grove Model for Implementing Evidence-Based Guidelines in Practice
  g. Iowa Model of Evidence-Based Practice
  h. Meta-analysis
  i. Meta-synthesis
  j. Mixed methods systematic review
  k. PICOS question
  l. Stetler Model of Research Utilization to Facilitate Evidence-Based Practice
 m. Systematic review
  n. Translational research

Definitions

_____ 1. A synthesis process of statistically pooling the results from previous quantitative studies using statistical analyses to determine the effect of an intervention or the strength of a relationship in a selected health-related area.

_____ 2. Clinical decision-making trees or figures nurses use when implementing research evidence in practice.

_____ 3. A structured, comprehensive synthesis of quantitative studies in a particular healthcare area or to address a practice problem to determine the best research evidence available for use in practice.

_____ 4. Highest quality research knowledge produced by the conduct and synthesis of numerous high-quality studies in a health-related area.

_____ 5. Patient care guidelines that are based on synthesized research findings from systematic reviews, meta-analyses, and extensive clinical trials; supported by consensus from recognized national experts; and affirmed by outcomes obtained by clinicians.

_____ 6. A format for initiating a research synthesis related to a clinical question that includes the following elements: population of interest, intervention needed for practice, comparison of interventions to determine best practice, outcomes needed for practice, and study designs.

_____ 7. This is a comprehensive framework to enhance the use of research evidence by nurses in their practice that includes the phases of preparation, validation, comparative evaluation/decision making, translation/application, and evaluation.

_____ 8. Synthesis of the findings from independent studies conducted with a variety of methods (quantitative, qualitative, and mixed methods) to determine the current knowledge in a selected healthcare area.

_____ 9. Designated sites by the Agency for Healthcare Research and Quality (AHRQ) for the development of research in designated areas and the translation of the evidence-based findings into clinical practice.

_____ 10. A process and product of systematically reviewing, compiling, and integrating qualitative study findings to expand understanding and develop a unique interpretation of the studies' findings in a selected health area.

_____ 11. A model developed in 1994 and revised in 2017 by a nursing collaborative that provides direction for the development of EBP in a clinical agency.

_____ 12. Type of research defined by the National Institutes of Health (NIH) as a methodology for promoting the use of basic scientific discoveries into practical applications.

_____ 13. Conscientious integration of best research evidence with nurses' clinical expertise and patients' circumstances and values in the delivery of quality, safe, cost-effective health care.

_____ 14. Framework developed by one of the authors of your text to promote the use of evidence-based guidelines in practice.

EXERCISE 2: LINKING IDEAS

Directions: Fill in the blanks with the appropriate word(s)/response(s).

1. List four benefits of developing an EBP for nursing.

a. _____

b. _____

c. _____

d. _____

2. Identify three sources you might access to keep current with the research literature.

a. _____

b. _____

c. _____

3. Identify two challenges to accomplishing EBP in nursing:

   a. _____

   b. _____

4. Identify two reasons why nursing lacks the research evidence needed for implementing an EBP:

   a. _____

   b. _____

5. The Iowa Model included triggering issues and opportunities to promote EBP in clinical agencies. Identify two of these triggers:

   a. _____

   b. _____

6. Identify and describe three ways that research findings might be translated or applied into nursing practice that were discussed related to Stetler's Model of Research Utilization to Facilitate Evidence-Based Practice:

   a. _____

   Description:_____

   b. _____

   Description:_____

   c. _____

   Description:_____

   _____

7. Identify three resources for locating research syntheses of nursing knowledge. (Hint: Review Table 13.1 in Chapter 13 of *Grove and Gray Understanding Nursing Research* 7th edition text.)

   a. _____

   b. _____

   c. _____

8. The evaluation phase of the Stetler Model of Research Utilization to Facilitate Evidence-Based Practice includes formal and informal measurement of outcomes for the following groups:

   a. _____

   b. _____

   c. _____

9. The comparative evaluation phase of Stetler's Model includes four parts: substantiating evidence, fit of the setting,

_____ , and _____ .

10. Identify the three options of the decision-making phase of Stetler's Model:

    a. _____

    b. _____

    c. _____

11. NIH developed funding awards for translational research to improve the

    _____.

12. In 1997, the AHRQ established 12 _____
    _____ to promote the conduct of research, development of evidence-based guidelines
    for practice, and the implementation of translational research.

Understanding Research Syntheses

Directions: Match the particular type of research synthesis with the appropriate strategies used to conduct these syntheses. Some of the answers include more than one type of research synthesis.

Types of Research Synthesis
a. Systematic review
b. Meta-analysis
c. Meta-synthesis
d. Mixed methods systematic review

Synthesis Strategies

_____   1. Review that includes syntheses of a variety of quantitative and qualitative study designs to determine the current knowledge about medication administration technologies and patient safety.

_____   2. Grey literature should be included in which types of research syntheses?

_____   3. The systematic compiling and integration of the results from qualitative studies to expand understanding and develop a unique interpretation of women's experiences related to losing a child.

_____   4. A structured, comprehensive synthesis of the research literature to determine the best research evidence available to address the following healthcare question: What are the best interventions to promote weight loss in adolescents? This synthesis might include meta-analysis and other types of research synthesis.

_____   5. The PICOS format (**P**opulation, **I**ntervention, **C**omparison, **O**utcomes, and **S**tudy designs) is used to generate a clinical question to direct these types of research synthesis.

_____   6. Meta-summary is the summarizing of findings across qualitative reports to identify knowledge in a selected area, and this summary is part of this research synthesis.

_____   7. One type of research synthesis might use only randomized controlled trials (RCTs) and meta-analyses as sources.

_____   8. Research synthesis that involves the statistical pooling of the results from previous studies into a single quantitative analysis that provides one of the highest levels of evidence about the effectiveness of music in promoting rest in an intensive care unit (ICU).

_____   9. Ancestry searches use citations in relevant studies to identify additional studies. Which of these research syntheses use ancestry searches?

_____ 10. The reports from this type of qualitative synthesis might be presented in different formats based on the knowledge developed and the perspective of the authors.

_____ 11. Multilevel synthesis and parallel synthesis are two different approaches that might be used in conducting this type of research synthesis.

_____ 12. A funnel plot might be developed to assess for biases in a group of studies when conducting this type of research synthesis.

_____ 13. The synthesis of qualitative studies to describe the experience of postpartum depression.

_____ 14. Publication and reporting biases can weaken the validity of what types of research synthesis?

_____ 15. A preferred reporting statement called PRISMA has been developed to promote consistency and quality in the development of these two types of research syntheses.

Application of the Phases of Stetler's Model

Directions: Match the phase in Stetler's Model with the appropriate description and/or example. Each phase is used only once and all phases are identified.

Phases

a. Preparation
b. Validation
c. Comparative evaluation/decision making
d. Translation/application
e. Evaluation

Descriptions

_____ 1. The phase in which nurses evaluate the feasibility of using the Braden Scale to prevent pressure ulcers in their clinical agency.

_____ 2. The phase in which nurses develop a formal protocol for treatment of stage IV pressure ulcers in older adults.

_____ 3. The first awareness of the existence of an exercise program for severely disabled children obtained from attending a research conference and reading the study and similar studies in research journals.

_____ 4. Research knowledge about prevention of hospitalized infections is synthesized and evaluated using specific criteria.

_____ 5. The incidence of hospital-acquired infections is examined following the implementation of a new protocol to prevent infections.

Application of the Iowa Model of Evidence-Based Practice

Directions: Match the steps in the Iowa Model with the appropriate description and/or example. Each step is used only once and all steps are included.

Steps

a. Trigger issues or opportunities
b. State a question or purpose
c. Assemble, appraise, and synthesize body of evidence
d. Design and pilot practice change
e. Integrate and sustain practice change
f. Disseminate results

Descriptions

_____   1. The nurses were provided support to continue the fall prevention program and the number and types of falls were monitored through the hospital quality improvement program.

_____   2. A systematic review was conducted with 15 RCTs and a meta-analysis to identify an effective fall prevention program for the medical unit.

_____   3. Nurses and their manager noted an increased fall rate on their medical unit for the last two months.

_____   4. The results of the fall prevention program were communicated to the unit nurses and hospital administration.

_____   5. The nurses piloted the fall prevention program on just their medical unit.

_____   6. What interventions are currently used to prevent patient falls in the hospital? Are there more effective evidence-based interventions to implement to decrease the patient fall rate?

Agency's Readiness for Evidence-Based Practice

Directions: Think about the clinical agency in which you are currently doing your clinical hours. Provide responses to the following questions and discuss them in class or on your class discussion board.

1. Are the agency's policies, protocols, algorithms, and guidelines based on research? (**Yes** or **No**) Provide a rationale for your answer.

   _____

   _____

2. If you answered "no" to the previous question, what is the basis of the policies, protocols, algorithms, or guidelines of your agency?

   _____

   _____

3. Who are the individuals identified for promoting EBP changes in this agency? (Record the job titles of those involved.)

   _____

   _____

4. Does the agency provide access to research publications for nurses? If so, provide some examples of these publications.

   _____

   _____

5. Does the agency have the goal of EBP? _____

   _____

6. Is the agency seeking Magnet status? What is the link of EBP to Magnet status? _____

   _____

   _____

   _____

7. Locate the following study:
   Friesen, M. A., Brady, J. M., Milligan, R., & Christensen, P. (2017). Findings from a pilot study: Bringing evidence-based practice to the bedside. *Worldviews on Evidence-Based Nursing, 14*(1), 22–34.
   This study might provide nurses guidance in promoting EBP in their clinical agency. What was the purpose of this study?

   _____

   _____

   _____

EXERCISE 3: WEB-BASED INFORMATION AND RESOURCES

Directions: Fill in the blanks below with the appropriate responses.

1. The Agency for Healthcare Research and Quality (AHRQ) National Guideline Clearinghouse at http://www.guidelines.gov provides numerous guidelines to manage nursing and other healthcare problems. On this website, identify where you can search for evidence-based guideline summaries by clinical specialty:

   _____

   _____

2. The Oncology Nursing Society website (http://ons.org) has a "Practice Resource" section that includes "Putting Research Evidence into Practice (PEP)." Find this site and locate the EBP guidelines for managing anxiety in patients with cancer:

   _____

   Was the EBP information on managing anxiety current? _____.

Provide a rationale for your answer: _____

_____

3. Cochrane Nursing Care Field (CNCF) is part of the Cochrane Collaboration and can be found at http://cncf.cochrane.org/. Using that website, identify the site for the Cochrane Resources in Nursing:

_____

4. Locate the Nursing Reference Center (NRC) website. Identify the location for the Patient Education Reference Center on this site:

_____

5. Locate the U.S. Preventive Services Task Force: Recommendations for Adults website: _____

_____

6. Search for the Healthy People 2020 website. Identify the location of this website: _____

_____

7. Identify the website for Genomics that is a new topic for Healthy People 2020 website: _____

_____

EXERCISE 4: CONDUCTING CRITICAL APPRAISALS TO BUILD AN EVIDENCE-BASED PRACTICE

Directions: Read and critically appraise the systematic review and meta-analysis of randomized controlled trials conducted by Boitor, Gélinas, Richard-Lalonde, and Thombs (2017). The critical appraisal guidelines for systematic reviews and meta-analyses are presented in Table 13.2 in your textbook, *Understanding Nursing Research*, 7th edition. The complete citation for this research synthesis follows:

Boitor, M., Gélinas, C., Richard-Lalonde, M., & Thombs, B. D. (2017). The effect of massage on acute postoperative pain in critically and acutely ill adults post-thoracic surgery: Systematic review and meta-analysis of randomized controlled trials. *Heart & Lung, 46*(5), 339–346.

You can locate this study in the Research Article Library on the Evolve website for *Understanding Nursing Research*, 7th edition, at http://evolve.elsevier.com/grove/understanding/. Read the synthesis report to answer the following questions.

1. What was the objective of the systematic review and meta-analysis, and was it clearly presented? _____

_____

_____

_____

_____

2. What format was used for reporting the meta-analysis? Is this a strength or weaknesses? Provide a rationale for your answer: _____

_____

_____

_____

3. Apply the PICOS format to this research synthesis:

Population:

_____

Intervention:

_____

Comparison of groups:

_____

_____

Outcomes:

_____

Study designs:

_____

4. Was the search of the research literature rigorous and clearly described? Provide a rationale to support your answer.

_____

_____

_____

_____

5a. How many total citations were retrieved?

_____

b. How many studies underwent full-text review?

_____

c. What was the final number of studies selected for the systematic review? _____

   d. Is a detailed discussion and flow chart provided to document the selection process for the studies to be included in the synthesis?

_____

_____

6. How was the quality of the selected studies for review assessed? _____

_____

_____

_____

7. Was a meta-analysis conducted as part of this systematic review? _____

8. What was the main conclusion of this systematic review about the effectiveness of massage in reducing postcardiac surgery pain?

_____

_____

9. Was massage found to be clinically significant in reducing pain in cardiac surgery patients? (**Yes** or **No**) Provide a rationale for your answer: _____

_____

_____

_____

Additional Evidence-Based Practice Projects

1. Conduct a project to promote EBP in a selected area of your practice. Use the following steps as a guide.

   a. Identify a clinical problem using the PICOS format that might be improved by using research knowledge in practice.

   b. Locate and review the research syntheses and studies in this problem area.

   c. Summarize what is known and not known regarding this problem.

   d. Select a model or theory to direct your use of research evidence in practice, such as the Stetler's Model of Research Utilization to Facilitate Evidence-Based Practice, or the Iowa Model of Evidence-Based Practice.

   e. Assess your agency's readiness to make the change.

   f. Provide education about the evidence-based change proposed to the nursing personnel, other health professionals, and administration.

   g. Implement the evidence-based change by a protocol, algorithm, or policy to be used in practice.

    h. Provide resources and emotional support to those persons involved in making the evidence-based change in practice.

    i. Develop evaluation strategies to determine the effects or outcomes of the evidence-based change on patient, provider, and agency.

    j. Evaluate over time to determine whether the evidence-based change should be continued. You might also extend the change to additional units or clinical agencies.

2. Use the Grove Model for Implementing Evidence-Based Guidelines to implement an evidence-based guideline from the Agency for Healthcare Research and Quality website in your practice.

    a. Identify a practice problem.

    b. Determine there is an evidence-based guideline to address the practice problem.

    c. Examine the quality of the evidence-based guideline.

    d. Integrate the evidence-based guideline with nurses' clinical expertise.

    e. Use the evidence-based guideline in practice.

    f. Monitor outcomes from use of the evidence-based guideline in practice.

    g. Refine the evidence-based guideline as needed.

14 Introduction to Additional Research Methodologies in Nursing: Mixed Methods and Outcomes Research

INTRODUCTION

You need to read Chapter 14 and then complete the following exercises. These exercises will assist you in learning relevant terms and in reading and comprehending published outcomes studies. The answers for these exercises are in the Answer Key at the back of the book.

EXERCISE 1: TERMS AND DEFINITIONS

Directions: Match each term below with its correct definition. Each term is used only once and all terms are defined.

Terms

a. Administrative databases
b. Clinical databases
c. Convergent concurrent design
d. Distal outcome
e. Explanatory sequential design
f. Exploratory sequential design
g. Mixed methods research
h. Nurses' roles in outcomes
i. Nursing Care Report Card

j. Nursing-sensitive patient outcomes
k. Outcomes research
l. Patient health outcomes
m. Pragmatism
n. Proximal outcome
o. Quality of care
p. Standard of care
q. Structures of care

Definitions

_____ 1. These outcomes are influenced by nursing care decisions and actions.

_____ 2. These outcomes are clearly interwoven into the entire care context and include the following: symptom control, reduced complications, functional status, knowledge of disease and its treatment, satisfaction with care, and cost of care.

_____ 3. A philosophy that supports developing studies to solve problems by whatever methods fit the problem or question.

_____ 4. An established field of health research that focuses on the end results of patient care.

_____ 5. Databases that are created by insurance companies, government agencies, and others not directly involved in providing patient care.

_____ 6. Have three subcomponents that include nurses' independent role functions, nurses' dependent role functions, and nurses' interdependent role functions.

_____ 7. Study designs that use both quantitative and qualitative methods.

_____ 8. An outcome that is close to the delivery of care.

_____ 9. A study design in which qualitative methods are implemented first with the researchers using the qualitative results to design a quantitative phase of the study.

_____ 10. This includes a group of indicators that could facilitate the benchmarking, or setting of a desired standard, that would allow comparisons of hospitals in terms of their nursing care quality.

_____ 11. The elements of organization and administration, as well as provider and patient characteristics that guide the processes of care.

_____ 12. A study design in which quantitative and qualitative methods are both used and the findings of each set of methods are used to corroborate the findings of the other.

_____ 13. A norm on which quality of care is judged, such as clinical guidelines, critical paths, and care maps.

_____ 14. An outcome that is removed from the care or a service received and might be more influenced by external (nontreatment) factors.

_____ 15. The degree to which health services for individuals and populations increase the likelihood of desired health outcomes and are consistent with current professional knowledge.

_____ 16. Databases that are created by providers such as hospitals, clinics, and healthcare professionals.

_____ 17. A study design in which a quantitative phase is followed by a qualitative phase and the qualitative results explain and expand the quantitative results.

EXERCISE 2: LINKING IDEAS

Key Ideas for Mixed Methods Research

1. What are the three types of mixed methods designs described in the chapter?

   a. _____

   b. _____

   c. _____

2. The _____ philosophy is often the foundation for mixed methods studies.

3. List two reasons why a mixed methods study may require more time to complete when compared to either a quantitative or qualitative study.

   a. _____

   _____

   b. _____

   _____

4. In the exploratory sequential mixed methods design, (**qualitative** or **quantitative**) data collection occurs first. _(Circle the correct answer.)_

5. What is another name for the convergent concurrent design? _____

6. Name five criteria by which mixed methods studies are critically appraised:

   a. _____

   b. _____

   c. _____

   d. _____

   e. _____

Key Ideas for Outcomes Research

Directions: Fill in the blanks in this section with the appropriate word(s)/ response(s).

1. A major theory dominating outcomes research was developed by _____.

2. Donabedian's cube (see Figure 14.5 in your textbook, *Understanding Nursing Research*, 7th edition) included which three aspects of health?

   a. _____

   b. _____

   c. _____

3. Donabedian identified three foci of evaluation in appraising quality. Identify these three foci and provide an example of each:

   a. _____

   b. _____

   c. _____

4. Nursing Role Effectiveness Model (see Figure 14.6 in your textbook) provided a framework for conceptualizing

   _____.

5. Nurses' independent role functions include

   _____

   _____.

6. Nurses' interdependent role functions include such actions as

   _____

   _____.

7. To evaluate an outcome as defined by Donabedian, the identified outcomes must be clearly linked to the process of care that caused the _____.

8. List three examples of standards of care:

   a. _____

   b. _____

   c. _____

9. **Heterogeneous** or **Homogeneous** samples are preferred in outcomes studies. *(Circle the correct answer.)*

10. From an outcomes research perspective, identify three questions nurse researchers might address in conducting outcomes studies:

   a. _____

   b. _____

   c. _____

11. What are two types of databases that are important sources of data for outcomes studies?

   a. _____

   b. _____

12. Statistical methods for outcomes studies focus on analysis of _____ and

   _____.

13. What are the three major questions used for critically appraising outcomes studies?

   a. _____

   b. _____

   c. _____

Mixed Methods Research Methodologies

Directions: Match each methodology below with its correct description. Each methodology is used at least once and may be used more than once.

Methodologies
a. Concurrent convergent design
b. Explanatory sequential design
c. Exploratory sequential design

Descriptions

_____   1. The researchers asked participants to report their pain level each day for 10 days using a visual analog scale with a possible range of scores from 0–100. The data were analyzed and used to categorize participants as low pain, medium pain, and high pain. During the qualitative phase, participants in each category were interviewed and asked to describe their pain. Themes from each group were compared and descriptions of each type of pain experience were created.

_____ 2. While developing the proposal for a study, a team of researchers identify that quantitative researchers studying self-care efficacy had reported conflicting findings. In order to increase self-care efficacy of persons newly diagnosed with type 1 diabetes, the researchers decide to administer a self-care efficacy instrument and ask participants whether they would be willing to participate in a focus group at a later time.

_____ 3. The researchers conducted a series of three interviews with 22 persons newly diagnosed with diabetes about the challenges to making lifestyle changes. During the same time, the researchers were collecting quantitative data about lifestyle changes from another group of persons newly diagnosed with diabetes. The qualitative and quantitative data were analyzed separately and then combined to provide a comprehensive description of making lifestyle changes related to diabetes.

_____ 4. A team of researchers evaluated instruments to measure symptom management of persons with multiple chronic illnesses. When they found none of the instruments were appropriate for their patients, they decided to conduct a mixed methods study. They conducted focus groups with their patients about symptom management. They analyzed the qualitative data and identified three themes. For each theme, they developed three to five items to measure symptom management using the focus group participants' words and phrases. The researchers then tested the instrument by administering the instrument to a national sample of persons with chronic illnesses.

_____ 5. A team of researchers recruit participants with early-stage heart failure for a mixed methods study and obtain informed consent. The participants are individually interviewed and then asked to complete a pencil-and-paper questionnaire on medication instructions and lifestyle changes before they leave.

Outcomes Research Methodologies

Directions: Match each methodology below with its correct description. Each methodology is used only once and all methodologies are described.

Methodologies
a. Population-based studies
b. Prospective cohort study
c. Retrospective cohort study
d. Secondary analysis
e. Standardized mortality ratio (SMR)

Descriptions

_____ 1. An epidemiological study in which the researcher identifies a group of people who have experienced a particular event for investigation, such as an infection following a surgical procedure.

_____ 2. The observed number of deaths are divided by the expected number of deaths and multiplied by 100.

_____ 3. Studies conducted within the context of the patients' community rather than the context of the medical system, such as the elderly individuals' physical and psychological functional levels in their homes.

_____ 4. An epidemiological study where researchers identify a group of people who are at risk for experiencing a particular event and then follow them over time to observe whether the event occurs, such as the incidence of health problems in morbidly obese individuals.

_____ 5. A study that involves any re-analysis of data or information collected by another researcher or organization, including analysis of data sets collected from a variety of sources.

EXERCISE 3: WEB-BASED INFORMATION AND RESOURCES

Mixed Methods Research

Directions: Search on the web for the following resources related to mixed methods research.

1. Find the document "Best Practices for Mixed Methods Research in the Health Sciences" on the website for the Office of Behavioral and Social Sciences Research, National Institute of Health. Provide the URL for the document:

    _____

2. AHRQ has published a document online about mixed methods research by Wisdom and Creswell (2013). Find the document "Mixed Methods: Integrating Quantitative and Qualitative Data Collection and Analysis While Studying Patient-Centered Medical Home Models." Provide the URL for the document:

    _____

3. Use the Wisdom and Creswell (2013) document to answer this question. Wisdom and Creswell (2013, p. 2) identified the goals of five mixed methods designs in the section, II. Uses of Mixed Methods Designs. One of the reasons given is to "Validate findings using quantitative and qualitative data sources." Provide two other reasons that are given by the authors:

    a. _____

    b. _____

Outcomes Research

Directions: Supply the full name for each organization acronym. Then, search the web to find these organizations and identify the website for each that discusses their contribution to outcomes research.

1. AHRQ

    Full name: _____

    Website: _____

2. ANA

    Full name: _____

    Website: _____

3. CALNOC

    Full name: _____

    Website: _____

4. NDNQI

    Full name: _____

    Website: _____

5. NINR

   Full name: _____

   Website: _____

6. NIC

   Full name: _____

   Website: _____

7. NQF

   Full name: _____

   Website: _____

8. ONS

   Full name: _____

   Website: _____

EXERCISE 4: CONDUCTING CRITICAL APPRAISALS TO BUILD AN EVIDENCE-BASED PRACTICE

Mixed Methods Research

Directions: The article used for the questions in this section is available as Appendix C. The citation is as follows:

Wendler, M., Smith, K., Ellenburg, W., Gill, R., Anderson, L., & Spiegel-Thayer, K. (2017). "To see with my own eyes": Experiences of family visits during phase 1 recovery. *Journal of PeriAnesthesia Nursing, 32*(1), 45–57.

Answer the following questions related to the study. Several aspects of this study have been critically appraised in previous study guide chapters. The open-ended questions will focus on the mixed methods aspects of the research report.

1. What was the purpose of the study?

   _____

   _____

   _____

   _____

2. Use the two questions about the study (Figure 14.1) to determine the mixed method study design.

   _____

3. Wendler et al. (2017) provided a discussion of how they increased the rigor of the qualitative component of study. For each statement from the article, identify the characteristic of rigor that was enhanced by these actions.

    a. "research results were presented to numerous audiences of post-anesthesia care unit (PACU) nurses, who expressed verbally their ability to implement similar changes in their own units" (Wendler et al., 2017, p. 51).

    _____

    b. "supported in the research results of the participants' own words" (Wendler et al., 2017, p. 51–52).

    _____

    c. "supported through triangulation of researchers and maintaining fidelity to the participants' own words" (Wendler et al., 2017, p. 51).

    _____

    d. "occurred through a careful description of the processes used to evaluate the quantitative and qualitative data" (Wendler et al., 2017, p. 51).

    _____

4. Write the research question that was answered by the qualitative component of the study.

    _____

    _____

5. What was the overarching theme of the qualitative results (Wendler et al., 2017, p. 55)?

    _____

    _____

6. For each study characteristic, identify whether it is a strength (**S**) or a weakness (**W**) and provide a rationale for your answer.

    _____

    _____ a. The title did not include or infer that the study was a mixed methods study.

    _____ b. The research team included a PhD-prepared nurse, two master's prepared nurses, and two student assistants.

    _____ c. A convenience sample was recruited.

    _____ d. Participants served as their own controls in the study.

    _____ e. The researchers provided information about the machine used to collect the data about vital signs.

    _____ f. The Cronbach alpha for the STAI was reported by the researchers.

    _____ g. The telephone interview was conducted with the patient and family member at the same time.

_____ h. Study findings were connected to the research framework, Roy's adaption theory (Wendler et al., 2017, p. 53).

_____ i. Based on the study findings, the researchers recommended offering family visits during phase I recovery to all surgical patients.

Outcomes Research

Directions: The article used for the questions in this section is available in an open-access journal. Open-access journals can be retrieved through an Internet search. The citation is as follows:

Dizon, M. P., Linos, E., Arron, S., Hills, N., & Chren, M. (2017). Comparing the quality of ambulatory surgical care for skin cancer in a Veterans Affairs clinic and a fee-for-service practice using clinical and patient-reported measures. *PLOS One, 17*(1), January 31, 2017. Retrieved on October 28, 2017, from http://journals.plos.org/plosone/article?id=10.1371/journal.pone.0153704

Answer the following questions related to this study.

1. What outcome research methodology was used by Dizon et al. (2017)? Give a rationale for your answer.

   _____

   _____

   _____

   _____

2. Using the text and Figure 1 in the article, identify the process and outcome measures used in the study. Clinical process measures were: _____

   _____

   _____

   _____

   Clinical and patient-reported outcomes were: _____

   _____

   _____

3. How was "time to treatment" defined? _____

   _____

   _____

4. What was the sample size of this study? Critically appraise the sample size of this study. _____

   _____

   _____

   _____

   _____

5. What was the setting for this study? Did the participants from the sites have the same demographic and treatment characteristics?

_____

_____

_____

_____

6. For each of these process measures, indicate which setting had the participants with that characteristic. Answer with **VA** for Veterans Affairs and **FFS** for fee-for-service.

   a. Longer time between biopsy and treatment _____

   b. More likely to use postoperative pain medicine _____

   c. More frequent follow-up with dermatology _____

7. What were the key findings from this study? They are summarized in the discussion section.

_____

_____

_____

_____

_____

8. Critically appraise the quality of this outcomes study. _____

_____

_____

_____

_____

_____

_____

Answer Key to Study Guide Exercises

CHAPTER 1—INTRODUCTION TO NURSING RESEARCH AND ITS IMPORTANCE IN BUILDING AN EVIDENCE-BASED PRACTICE

EXERCISE 1: TERMS AND DEFINITIONS

Acquiring Knowledge and Research Methods

1. f	9. l
2. h	10. c
3. d	11. i
4. j	12. k
5. n	13. g
6. b	14. o
7. p	15. a
8. e	16. m

Evidence-Based Practice Terms

1. e
2. b
3. a
4. d
5. c

Synthesizing Research Evidence

1. e
2. a
3. d
4. c
5. b

EXERCISE 2: LINKING IDEAS

How Research Influences Practice

1. Description involves identifying the nature and attributes of nursing phenomena. Descriptive knowledge generated through research can be used to identify and describe what exists in nursing practice, to discover new information, and to classify information of use in the discipline.
   Examples: a. Identifying the signs and symptoms for making the nursing diagnosis of acute pain. b. Describing women who are at risk for acute myocardial infarction. c. Describing the incidence and spread of infection in healthcare agencies.

2. Explanation focuses on identifying and clarifying the strength and nature of relationships among variables or concepts relevant for practice.
   Example: Determining the relationships of the health-related quality-of-life domains (physical functioning, role limitations, social functioning, general health, and energy fatigue) and depressive symptoms among seropositive African Americans. This correlational study was conducted by Coleman (2017), and the study can be found in the Article Library for the Grove and Gray (2019) *Understanding Nursing Research*, 7th edition, at http://evolve.elsevier.com/grove/understanding.

3. Prediction involves estimating the probability of a specific outcome in a given situation.
   Example: Research findings predict that family cardiac history, pack years of smoking (number of packs smoked per day times the number of years smoking), abnormal lipid levels, hypertension, and obesity are linked to an increased incidence of coronary heart disease. With predictive knowledge, nurses can identify the risk levels of patients for coronary heart disease.

4. Control is the ability to manipulate a situation to produce the desired outcomes in practice. Therefore, nurses could prescribe certain interventions to help patients and families achieve quality outcomes.
   Example: You would prescribe the use of warm, not cold, applications for the resolution of normal saline intravenous infiltrations. Stress reduction exercises might be prescribed as an additional treatment for high blood pressure. Health promotion programs need to be implemented in healthcare agencies to reduce burnout and improve job satisfaction for nurses.

Historical Events Influencing Nursing Research

1. Florence Nightingale
2. *Nursing Research*
3. You might list any three of the following journals or identify other research journals published in nursing:
   Advances in Nursing Science
   Applied Nursing Research
   Biological Research for Nursing
   Clinical Nursing Research
   Journal of Nursing Scholarship
   Nursing Research
   Nursing Science Quarterly
   Qualitative Health Research
   Research in Nursing & Health
   Scholarly Inquiry for Nursing Practice
   Western Journal of Nursing Research
4. Sigma Theta Tau
5. 1985
6. National Institute of Nursing Research (NINR)
7. International North American Nursing Diagnosis Association (NANDA-I)
8. Agency for Healthcare Research and Quality (AHRQ)
9. *Healthy People 2020*
10. American Nurses Credentialing Center

Acquiring Knowledge in Nursing

1. You could have identified any of the following ways of acquiring knowledge in nursing. Some possible examples of each way of acquiring nursing knowledge are provided.
   a. Tradition: giving a report on hospitalized patients in the same way over time or organizing the care provided to the patients, such as bathing, in a standard way over years.
   b. Authority: expert clinical nurses, educators, and authors of articles or books.
   c. Borrowing: using knowledge from medicine, psychology, or sociology in nursing practice.
   d. Trial and error: positioning a patient in different ways to reduce his or her discomfort during an intramuscular injection or trying different interventions to help patients sleep in the Intensive Care Unit (ICU).
   e. Personal experience: obtaining knowledge by being in a clinical agency and providing care to patients and families.
   f. Role modeling: a new graduate in an internship being mentored by an expert nurse who models excellent clinical practice behavior.
   g. Intuition: knowing that a patient's condition is deteriorating, but having limited concrete data to support this feeling or hunch.

   h. Reasoning: reasoning from the general to the specific or deductive reasoning; reasoning from the specific to the general or inductive reasoning.
   i. Research: quantitative, qualitative, mixed methods, and outcomes research conducted to generate nursing knowledge.
2. personal experience
3. a. novice
   b. advanced beginner
   c. competent
   d. proficient
   e. expert
4. Research, empirical, or scientific
5. intuition
6. Deductive reasoning
7. You might identify any of the following important outcomes examined in outcomes research:
   (a) patient health status (signs, symptoms, functional status, morbidity, mortality); (b) patient satisfaction; (c) costs related to health care; (d) quality of care; (e) quality of care provider; (f) provider satisfaction; and (g) access to care by patients and families.
8. Sethares and Asselin (2017) conducted a mixed methods study as indicated by the following study excerpt.
   "The purpose of this exploratory study was to test the acceptability and effect of a guided reflective intervention on self-care maintenance and management scores in persons with HF. A one-group mixed method pre-test/post-test exploratory design, using qualitative and quantitative approaches, was used to answer the following research questions: 1. How do heart failure patients describe their self-care in general and during periods of exacerbation? 2. What is the effect of a guided reflection intervention on self-care maintenance and management scores? 3. To what extent is guided reflection useful and acceptable to heart failure patients in gaining insights into self-care decisions?" (Sethares & Asselin, 2017, p. 193).
   Rationale: Authors called the study a mixed methods study that included qualitative and quantitative approaches.

Linking Research Methods to Types of Research

1. b
2. b
3. a
4. b
5. a
6. a
7. a
8. b
9. a and b

Nurses' Roles in Research

1. a
2. d and/or e
3. a, b, c, d, and e
4. d and/or e
5. b, c, d, and/or e
6. a, b, and/or c
7. c, d, and e
8. b and/or c
9. e
10. d and e

Determining the Strength of Levels of Research Evidence

Rank order of the levels of research evidence is
4, 1, 3, 2, 6, 5.

EXERCISE 3: WEB-BASED INFORMATION AND RESOURCES

1. The current mission of the National Institute of Nursing Research (NINR, 2017) is to "promote and improve the health of individuals, families, communities, and populations. The Institute supports and conducts clinical and basic research and research training on health and illness across the lifespan to build the scientific foundation for clinical practice, prevent disease and disability, manage and eliminate symptoms caused by illness, and improve palliative and end-of-life care" (NINR website: https://www.ninr.nih.gov/aboutninr/ninr-mission-and-strategic-plan).
2. https://www.guidelines.gov
3. https://guidelines.gov/summaries/summary/48192/2014-evidencebased-guideline-for-the-management-of-high-blood-pressure-in-adults-report-from-the-panel-members-appointed-to-the-eighth-joint-national-committee-jnc-8?q=hypertension+in+adults/
4. https://www.healthypeople.gov/
5. https://www.healthypeople.gov/2020/topics-objectives/topic/Adolescent-Health
6. http://qsen.org/competencies/pre-licensure-ksas/
7. Evidence-Based Practice (EBP) Competency: "Integrate best current evidence with clinical expertise and patient/family preferences and values for delivery of optimal health care." This website also includes the knowledge, skills, and attitudes (KSAs) for the EBP competency.

EXERCISE 4: CONDUCTING CRITICAL APPRAISALS TO BUILD AN EVIDENCE-BASED PRACTICE

Research Methods

1. c
2. b
3. a

Researchers' Credentials

1. Donna Hallas has a PhD and is a certified pediatric nurse practitioner (PNP), which was identified through an Internet search. She is the director of the PNP program at New York University Rory Meyers College of Nursing. Dr. Hallas has a previous publication and two international presentations with Mary Koslap-Petraco focused on social-emotional development of toddlers that were cited in the reference list. Dr. Koslap-Petraco has a DNP and is also a certified PNP. National certification as a PNP requires current practice as nurse practitioner (NP). Dr. Koslap-Petraco is the coordinator of child health at the Suffolk County Department of Health and also has a faculty position at Long Island University. An Internet search of Dr. Jason Fletcher identified that he has a PhD in Applied Economics and is a Professor of Public Affairs and a Faculty Affiliate of the Institute for Research on Poverty at New York University. These three authors demonstrate strong educational, research, and clinical expertise for conducting this study. The study was supported by funding from the New York University Research Fund. The university funding indicates that the study was reviewed by research experts who chose to financially support the study.
2. Alyssa Erikson is PhD-prepared and an assistant professor in the School of Nursing at the University of California, San Francisco. Dr. Davies is also PhD-prepared and has previous publications cited in the reference list for this study. Her area of expertise is palliative care and she has 78 publications during her career. These authors demonstrate educational and research expertise to conduct this study. The clinical expertise is unclear when viewing the websites of Dr. Erikson and Dr. Davies. This study was supported by the Betty Irene Moore Predoctoral Fellowship at the University of California, San Francisco. This study was probably developed from Dr. Erikson's dissertation.
3. Dr. Wendler is PhD-prepared and nationally certified in her clinical area of expertise. She is the Director of Nursing Research and Academic Partnerships at Memorial Medical Center in Springfield, Illinois. Dr. Wendler had a previous study cited in the reference list. Katherine Smith has a master's in nursing and is a family NP. She was formerly a charge nurse at Memorial Medical Center. Wanda Ellenburg is also master's-prepared and a former nurse manager at Memorial Medical Center. Rita Gill, Lea Anderson, and Kim Spiegel-Thayer are registered nurses with Bachelor of Science in Nursing (BSN) preparation, who currently or formerly worked at Memorial Medical Center.

Dr. Wendler has educational, research, and clinical expertise to conduct this study. The other authors have clinical and educational expertise to collaborate in this study, with Dr. Wendler as the primary investigator. PhD-prepared nurses are encouraged to include other nurses in their research projects to expand their exposure to research activities. This study was funded in part by a grant from Illinois Society of PeriAnesthesia Nursing and also by the Memorial Medical Center Foundation. These grants indicate the study was reviewed by research experts and financially supported by a local organization and medical center.

Study Titles and Abstracts

1. Title: Hallas et al. (2017) titled their study "Social-emotional development of toddlers: Randomized controlled trial [RCT] of an office-based intervention". The title clearly identifies the study population as toddlers and indicates the type of study conducted, a RCT. RCT is a strong experimental study that focuses on the testing of an intervention. The title also identifies the focus of the study, which is examining the effects of an office-based intervention on the social-emotional development of toddlers. This is a significant area of research conducted to improve the health and well-being of toddlers and their mothers. The title included all the expected elements.

2. Abstract: The abstract for the Hallas et al. (2017) study concisely and clearly identified the following areas of the study: *Design and Methods*, *Results*, and *Conclusions*. The *Purpose* identified in the abstract is really the significance of the research problem for this study. The study purpose is provided in the *Design and Methods* section, which might confuse readers. The framework for the study should have been mentioned in the abstract. The specific study design, measurement method, and intervention were clearly addressed in the abstract. The results of the study indicated that both the treatment and control groups significantly improved, which is discussed in more detail in the study. The conclusions are acceptable but additional research with a larger sample is needed before the effectiveness of the intervention can be determined. The abstract would have been clearer if the purpose had been correctly identified.

Critical Appraisal of the Titles and Abstracts of Studies on Research Course Discussion Board

Put your critical appraisals of the titles and abstracts for the Erikson and Davies (2017) and Wendler et al. (2017) studies on the discussion board for your research course

and review the comments of other students. Clarify any questions with your faculty.

CHAPTER 2—INTRODUCTION TO QUANTITATIVE RESEARCH

EXERCISE 1: TERMS AND DEFINITIONS

1.	l	11.	m
2.	s	12.	n
3.	a	13.	f
4.	d	14.	t
5.	r	15.	o
6.	c	16.	g
7.	h	17.	e
8.	k	18.	i
9.	q	19.	p
10.	j	20.	b

EXERCISE 2: LINKING IDEAS

Control in Quantitative Research

1. highly controlled
2. descriptive and correlational
3. quasi-experimental and experimental
4. experimental
5. nonrandom or nonprobability; random or probability
6. natural
7. highly controlled
8. experimental
9. partially controlled
10. quasi-experimental and experimental

Steps of the Research Process

1. problem-solving process; nursing
2. Step 1: Research problem and purpose
   Step 2: Literature review
   Step 3: Research framework
   Step 4: Research objectives, questions, or hypotheses
   Step 5: Study variables
   Step 6: Research design
   Step 7: Population and sample
   Step 8: Methods of measurement
   Step 9: Data collection
   Step 10: Data analysis and results
   Step 11: Interpretation of research outcomes: Determining study findings, identifying study limitations, exploring the significance of the findings, forming conclusions, generalizing the findings, considering the implications for nursing, and suggesting further studies.

3. You could identify any of the following assumptions or other assumptions you have noted in research reports.
   a. People want to assume control of their own health and manage their health problems.
   b. Stress should be avoided.
   c. Health is a priority for most people.
   d. People who live in poor areas feel underserved for health care.
   e. Attitudes can be measured with a scale.
   f. Most measurable attitudes are held strongly enough to direct behavior.
   g. Health professionals view health care in a manner different from laypersons.
   h. Human biological and chemical factors show less variation than do cultural and social factors.
   i. People operate on the basis of cognitive information.
   j. Increased knowledge about an event lowers anxiety about the event.
   k. Receipt of health care at home is preferable to receipt of care in an institution.
4. You could identify any of the following reasons for conducting a pilot study:
   a. To determine whether the proposed study is feasible (e.g., Are the study participants available? Does the researcher have the time and money to conduct the study?)
   b. To develop or refine a research treatment or intervention
   c. To develop a protocol for the implementation of an intervention
   d. To identify problems with the design
   e. To determine whether the sample is representative of the population or whether the sampling technique is effective
   f. To examine the reliability and validity of the measurement methods to be used in a study
   g. To develop or refine data collection instruments
   h. To refine the data collection and analysis plan
   i. To give the researcher experience with the study participants, setting, methodology, and methods of measurement
   j. To try out data analysis techniques
5. limitations

Reading Research Reports

1. You could identify any of the following nursing research journals.
   a. *Advances in Nursing Science*
   b. *Applied Nursing Research*
   c. *Biological Research for Nursing*
   d. *Clinical Nursing Research*
   e. *Journal of Nursing Measurement*
   f. *Journal of Nursing Scholarship*
   g. *International Journal of Nursing Studies*
   h. *International Journal of Nursing Terminologies and Classifications*
   i. *Nursing Research*
   j. *Nursing Science Quarterly*
   k. *Qualitative Nursing Research*
   l. *Research in Nursing & Health*
   m. *Scholarly Inquiry for Nursing Practice*
   n. *Western Journal of Nursing Research*
   o. *Worldviews on Evidence-Based Nursing*
2. Look in clinical journals and see which ones have several research articles in each issue. You might have identified any of the following nursing clinical journals:
   a. *Geriatric Nursing*
   b. *Oncology Nursing Forum*
   c. *Nephrology Nursing*
   d. *Issues in Comprehensive Pediatric Nursing*
   e. *Journal of Transcultural Nursing*
   f. *Heart & Lung*
   g. *Journal of Nursing Education*
   h. *Birth*
   i. *Nursing Diagnosis*
   j. *Public Health Nursing*
   k. *The Diabetes Educator*
   l. *Maternal-Child Nursing Journal*
   m. *Journal of Nursing Education*
   n. *Journal of Pediatric Nursing*
   o. *Archives of Psychiatric Nursing*
3. a. Introduction
   b. Methods
   c. Results
   d. Discussion
4. You might have identified any of the following that are included in the methods section of a research report.
   a. Design
   b. Sample
   c. Setting
   d. Informed consent process
   e. Review of the study by institutional review boards
   f. Methods of measurement
   g. Data collection process
   h. Usually identifies the data analysis techniques to be conducted
   i. The methods section also includes the intervention if that is applicable to the type of study being conducted, such as for quasi-experimental and experimental studies.
5. You might have identified any of the following elements of the discussion section of a research report.
   a. Major findings
   b. Link of findings to previous study findings

c.   Limitations of the study
d.   Conclusions drawn from the findings
e.   Generalization of the study findings
f.   Implications of the findings for nursing
g.   Recommendations for further research
6.   introduction
7.   theoretical and empirical
8.   skimming, comprehending, and analyzing
9.   identifying and understanding the steps of the research process
10. determining the value of the research report's content by examining the quality and completeness of the steps of the research process and the links among these steps

Types of Quantitative Research

1.	c	9.	d
2.	a	10.	b
3.	b	11.	c or d
4.	a	12.	a
5.	c	13.	c
6.	d	14.	b
7.	b	15.	c
8.	a		

EXERCISE 3: WEB-BASED INFORMATION AND RESOURCES

1.   The National Human Genome Research Institute (NHGRI) is the name of the organization focused on human genome research in the US. The website for the institute is: https://www.genome.gov/
The funding website of NHGRI is: https://www.genome.gov/12010633/overview-of-the-extramural-research-program/
Genomic research began with the Human Genome Project (HGP).
2.   The NINR website is: https://www.ninr.nih.gov/. The "Research Highlights" are found on the following website: https://www.ninr.nih.gov/researchandfunding/researchhighlights
3.   The website presenting the reports funded by the AHRQ is: https://www.ahrq.gov/research/findings/index.html

EXERCISE 4: CONDUCTING CRITICAL APPRAISALS TO BUILD AN EVIDENCE-BASED PRACTICE

Type of Quantitative and/or Qualitative Research

1.   d. (Because randomized controlled trials are usually considered experimental studies. However, c. Quasi-experimental research could also be considered correct.)

2.   f. (Grounded theory research method in which the goal is to develop a theory that offers an explanation about the main concern of the population [nurses] and how that concern is resolved or processed.)
3.   a and g. ("This was a descriptive, single-group, mixed methods study" [Wendler et al., 2017, p. 45] that included descriptive quantitative and exploratory-descriptive qualitative methods.)

Type of Setting

1.   b. The Hallas et al. (2017) study was conducted in five pediatric primary healthcare offices and clinics. The offices and clinics were partially controlled for the implementation of the intervention DVDs and the collection of data with the Toddler Care Questionnaire and Brigance Toddler Screen.
2.   a. Erikson and Davies (2017, p. 43) reported the following about their study setting: "Interested RNs emailed or phoned the PI [principle investigator] to schedule a mutually convenient time and place to meet for an interview, most often in a private area at their workplace before or after their shift." The setting for this study was natural since it was a convenient place selected by the study participants and involved no control by the researchers.
3.   b. The Wendler et al. (2017) study was conducted in two settings: (1) a postanesthesia care unit (PACU) staffed by experienced registered nurses and (2) the family waiting area just outside the PACU doors staffed by hospital volunteers. Both settings would be considered partially controlled since they are structured and managed by hospital personnel.

Type of Research Conducted (Applied or Basic)

1.   a
2.   a

CHAPTER 3—INTRODUCTION TO QUALITATIVE RESEARCH

EXERCISE 1: TERMS AND DEFINITIONS

General Terms

1.	f	10.	e
2.	p	11.	b
3.	k	12.	i
4.	r	13.	q
5.	a	14.	g
6.	j	15.	c
7.	o	16.	l
8.	h	17.	m
9.	n	18.	d

Definitions Related to Ethnography

1. d
2. f
3. g
4. e
5. b
6. a
7. c

Definitions in Your Own Words

1. Observation is gathering data by being in specific environments and situations and using all of your senses to notice and record details.
2. Coding is assigning a label to a key phrase or sentence in a transcript. The codes are synthesized into themes.
3. Researcher–participant relationship is the communication and trust that connects the researcher and the participants and through which data are produced.

EXERCISE 2: LINKING IDEAS

People and Their Contributions to Qualitative Research

1. b
2. e
3. c
4. a
5. d

Qualitative Research Methodology

1. dwell
2. native
3. field notes
4. saturation
5. prompts

Approaches to Qualitative Research

1. E
2. P
3. EDQ
4. G
5. E
6. EDQ
7. P
8. G

EXERCISE 3: WEB-BASED INFORMATION AND RESOURCES

1. Although answers may vary, the table includes commonly found descriptions. Here are some websites where this information can be found.
   https://explorable.com/quantitative-and-qualitative-research
   http://atlasti.com/quantitative-vs-qualitative-research/
   https://www.slideshare.net/alirezahajarian/what-is-the-difference-and-similarity-between-qualitative-and-quantitative-research
   http://yourspace.minotstateu.edu/laurie.geller/QualitativeQuantitativeTable.pdf

Methodological Element	Qualitative	Quantitative
Data	Words	Numbers
How will findings be used?	To understand participant's perspective	To generalize findings to population
Perspective	Subjective	Objective
Characteristics of rigor	Truth, credibility	Reliability, validity, study control, type of design
Methods	Evolving methods	Predetermined methods
Size of sample	Fewer participants—more data from each	More subjects—specific, preset data collected
Relationship between researcher and participants	Researcher influences the method and the data collected	Researcher remains distant so can be objective

2. Information about the Chin (2017) study

Study Characteristic	Answer
Country/state in which the study was conducted.	Massachusetts, United States
Identify the qualitative approach used (phenomenology, grounded theory, exploratory-descriptive qualitative, ethnography research).	Exploratory-descriptive qualitative study
Identify the human experience or topic of the study.	Acute exacerbations of chronic obstructive pulmonary disease (COPD), symptoms and symptom patterns, delaying treatment
Describe the sample, including the total number, gender, reason for hospitalization, mean age, and ethnicity of the majority of the participants.	14 participants (5 males and 9 females) who were hospitalized for acute exacerbations of COPD. The mean age was 66.21 years and 11 of the 14 were white.
How were the data collected?	In-depth, semi-structured interviews using an interview guide the researcher developed to be consistent with the theoretical framework, Common Sense Model of Illness Representation (Leventhal, Meyer, & Nerenz, 1980)

EXERCISE 4: CONDUCTING CRITICAL APPRAISALS TO BUILD AN EVIDENCE-BASED PRACTICE

1. The purpose of the study was to "describe how pediatric nurses defined boundaries and present a theoretical conceptualization of the identified process for managing boundaries, entitled maintaining integrity" (p. 43).
2. The qualitative method used was grounded theory because it "focuses on processes and enables development of a theory or theoretical conceptualization" (p. 43). This method was appropriate because it matched the purpose of the study.
3. Maintaining integrity
4. a. 8
   b. 15.69 years
   c. 1 participant was Black.
5. Data were collected through interviews "using a semi-structured interview guide" (p. 42).
6. Yes, the interview questions provided the participants an opportunity to describe their work, stresses at work, and relationships with patients and families. These questions generated data that was relevant to the study purpose.
7. Yes. The data analysis and interpretation processes were consistent with the philosophical orientation of grounded theory, provided findings that were relevant to the study problem and purpose. The statement of the research problem was that "little is known about how nurses manage professional and personal boundaries within the context of PPC [pediatric palliative care]" (Erikson & Davies, 2017, p. 43).
8. Yes. Your answer may be any one of the themes of the study with an example of the quotation provided related to the theme. The themes were "personal and professional boundaries" (p. 44); "maintaining integrity" (p. 45); "behaving professionally" (p. 46); "connecting personally" (p. 46); "threatened integrity" (p. 46); " compromised integrity" (p.47); and "integrity restored" (p. 47).
9. a. Professional and personal
   b. Connecting personally/Behaving professionally
   c. 1) Advocating for self
      2) Taking time for self
      3) Focusing on self
10. Wendler et al. (2017) collected the qualitative data through telephone interviews with the patients and the family members who visited them in the postanesthesia care unit (PACU).
11. 243 secondary codes and 14 categories (p. 51)
12. The categories included "anticipation"; "anxiety"; "communication"; "glad surgery is over"; "hospitality"; "long-term relationships"; "PACU characteristics"; "patient experiences"; "presence"; "relief"; "'to see with my own eyes'"; "visit characteristics, outcomes, and recommendations"; and "wait: characteristics" (pp. 54–55).
    The example is a correct answer if it matches the quotation provided in Table 4.

CHAPTER 4—EXAMINING ETHICS IN NURSING RESEARCH

EXERCISE 1: TERMS AND DEFINITIONS

1. f
2. a
3. i
4. k
5. j
6. e
7. m
8. c
9. o
10. g
11. d
12. n
13. h
14. b
15. l

EXERCISE 2: LINKING IDEAS

1. a. Disclosure of essential study information to the subject
    b. Comprehension of this information by the subject
    c. Competency of the subject to give consent
    d. Voluntary consent by the subject to participate in the study
2. You might have identified any five of the following general information requirements of a study consent form.
    a. Purpose and procedures of the research study
    b. Length of the subject's involvement
    c. Benefits and risks or discomforts
    d. Compensation, if any, for research-related injury
    e. Disclosure of alternative treatments if available
    f. Confidentiality of records
    g. Contact persons
    h. Right to refuse or withdraw without loss of benefit
3. Voluntary
4. diminished autonomy
5. institutional review boards (IRBs)
6. a. Exempt from review
    b. Expedited review
    c. Full review
7. Breach of confidentiality. Note that raw data should not have subjects' names included. Researchers typically use subject numbers rather than names to help maintain confidentiality. Only approved members of the research team should have access to raw data. Additionally, extra care should be taken to ensure confidentiality of sensitive or personally damaging information such as drug use.
8. The type of review is determined by the IRB of the agency where the study is to be conducted.
9. Full review
10. Possible answers include:
    a. Fabrication of research results and recording or reporting them
    b. Falsification of research by manipulating research materials, equipment or processes
    c. Falsification of research by changing, or omitting data or results
    d. Plagiarism by using another person's ideas, processes, results or words without giving proper credit
    e. Duplicate publication which is publishing the study in more than one journal
11. Office of Research Integrity (ORI)
12. Yes, research misconduct is a current area of concern in nursing. Rationale may include recent plagiarism in published articles, research misconduct that lead to a retraction in the journal of publication, or reports of misconduct from the Office of Research Integrity. A duplicate publication of the same study without citing previous publications of the study is a common type of misconduct in nursing and medicine. The need to always be vigilant to prevent or identify misconduct in nursing research is another possible answer.
13. Yes. An increasing number of animals are being used by nurse scientists to generate basic research knowledge for the profession.
14. Office of Laboratory Animal Welfare (OLAW)
15. Association for Assessment and Accreditation of Laboratory Animal Care International (AAALAC International) formerly known as American Association for Accreditation of Laboratory Animal Care (AAALAC).

Historical Events, Ethical Codes, and Regulations

1. b
2. c
3. d
4. b
5. c
6. a
7. d
8. b
9. a
10. c

Ethical Principles

1. c
2. a
3. b and c
4. b and c
5. a and c

Federal Regulations Influencing the Conduct of Research

Review Box 4.2 for a summary of these regulations.

1. a
2. c
3. a
4. b
5. c

Ethics of Published Studies

1. e
2. b
3. f
4. c, a
5. d

EXERCISE 3: WEB-BASED INFORMATION AND RESOURCES

The following websites provide the location of the information requested for each question in this section. Search these websites and identify relevant information related to the ethical conduct of research.

1. https://www.hhs.gov/ohrp/regulations-and-policy/regulations/common-rule/index.html
2. https://www.hhs.gov/ohrp/regulations-and-policy/belmont-report/index.html
3. https://www.fda.gov/ScienceResearch/SpecialTopics/RunningClinicalTrials/default.htm
4. https://www.hhs.gov/hipaa/for-professionals/special-topics/research/index.html
5. https://ori.hhs.gov/case_summary
6. https://grants.nih.gov/grants/olaw/olaw.htm

EXERCISE 4: CONDUCTING CRITICAL APPRAISALS TO BUILD AN EVIDENCE-BASED PRACTICE

1. Hallas et al. (2017) indicated that IRB approval and informed consent for the mother–toddler dyads were obtained. Eligible potential participants were invited to participate in the study and "Each mother who volunteered to participate in the study provided written informed consent prior to enrollment in the study" (p. 35). This statement indicates that the researchers obtained informed consent from the study participants and specified the type of consent. The researchers also addressed assent since the toddlers in the participating mother–toddler dyads were children. "If a toddler refused to participate in assessment activities on the Brigance Toddler screen, this behavior would be considered refusal of toddler assent per IRB study approval, and the toddler and mother were excluded as study participants" (p. 35). Randomization assured that placement in either the control or intervention group was fair. In order to minimize risk the control group was provided with usual care for the population, which in this case was a "standardized DVD on toddler nutrition" (p. 35). This study appears to be ethical because the risks are minimal and the benefits are strong, resulting in a positive benefit-risk ratio.

2. Erikson and Davies (2017) indicated that IRB approval and informed consent were obtained. "Approval to conduct the study was obtained from the institutional review boards at the major university with which the researchers were affiliated and at each study site" (p. 43). "Interested RNs emailed or phoned the PI [principle investigator] to schedule a mutually convenient time and place to meet for an interview, most often in a private area at their workplace before or after their shift. Consent was obtained at this time" (p. 43). The information regarding informed consent could have been presented in greater detail and with greater clarity. The use of "at this time" (p. 43) after a phrase that discussed an initial e-mail/phone call as well as the interview made it difficult to decipher at which point the consent occurred. Additionally, the researchers did not specify if written or verbal consent was obtained. Interviews carry minimal risk, but researchers should acknowledge the risk of emotional distress during the interview as well as plans to minimize distress if such distress occurs. This study appears to be ethical because the risks are minimal and benefits from the knowledge create a positive benefit-risk ratio.

3. Wendler et al. (2017) indicated that IRB approval and informed consent were obtained. The "study was approved by the community institutional review board before the onset of the study" (p. 47). "In all cases, consent was completed before the day of the surgery" (p. 48). The information regarding informed consent could have been presented in greater detail. The researcher could have provided the process for informed consent and if a written consent was obtained. Although the intervention carried minimal risk, the researchers should have provided a plan to reduce risk and actions if any negative consequences occurred. This study appears to be ethical because the risks are minimal and the potential benefits are strong, resulting in a positive benefit-risk ratio.

CHAPTER 5—EXAMINING RESEARCH PROBLEMS, PURPOSES, AND HYPOTHESES

EXERCISE 1: TERMS AND DEFINITIONS

1.	g	7.	e
2.	i	8.	b
3.	f	9.	a
4.	d	10.	c
5.	j	11.	h
6.	k		

Types of Hypotheses

1.	f	5.	b
2.	e	6.	c
3.	h	7.	g
4.	d	8.	a

EXERCISE 2: LINKING IDEAS

Research Problem and Purpose

1. a. variables or concepts
   b. population
   c. setting
2. You might have identified any of the following or thought of another relevant reason:
   a. has an impact on or is applied in nursing practice
   b. expands previous research
   c. improves understanding of a problem by developing theory
   d. adds knowledge to current nursing research priorities
   e. related to a health problem that affects a large number of people.
3. You might have identified any of the following agencies or organizations: National Institute for Nursing Research (NINR), Agency for Healthcare Research and Quality (AHRQ), Healthy People 2020, World Health Organization (WHO), American Association of Critical-Care Nurses (AACN), or Oncology Nursing Society (ONS). You might have identified other national nursing and healthcare professional organizations that have research priorities identified online or in publications.
4. a. researchers' expertise, which focuses on educational preparation, research previously conducted, and clinical experiences
   b. financial commitment
   c. availability of study participants, facility, and equipment
   d. study's ethical considerations
5. significance

Understanding Hypotheses

1. b, c, d, g
2. a, c, e, g
3. b, c, d, g
4. a, e, g, h
5. b, d, g, h
6. b, c, e, f
7. a, c, d, g
8. b, d, g, h
9. a, c, e, g
10. b, e, f, h
11. You could state the directional hypothesis in either of the following ways:
    a. Increased age, decreased family support, and decreased health status are related to decreased self-care abilities in nursing home residents.
    b. Decreased age, increased family support, and increased health status are related to increased self-care abilities in nursing home residents.
12. Patients with chronic low-back pain receiving low-back massage experience no difference in their perceptions of low-back pain from those receiving no massage.

Identifying Types of Study Variables

1. a	9. a
2. c	10. c
3. b	11. b
4. a	12. c
5. a or b	13. b
6. a	14. b
7. b	15. a
8. b	16. c

Understanding Study Variables

1. b
2. c
3. d
4. a
5. b
6. d

EXERCISE 3: WEB-BASED INFORMATION AND RESOURCES

1. The website is https://www.cdc.gov/
2. The website is https://www.cdc.gov/violenceprevention/childabuseandneglect/index.html
3. The website is https://www.ninr.nih.gov/
4. Nursing research develops knowledge to build the scientific foundation for clinical practice, prevent disease and disability, manage and eliminate symptoms caused by illness, and enhance end-of-life and palliative care (NINR, 2017).
5. a. The American Academy of Pediatrics includes the following website focused on the immunization schedule for children and adolescents less than 18 years of age: https://www.aap.org/en-us/advocacy-and-policy/aap-health-initiatives/immunizations/Pages/Immunization-Schedule.aspx
   b. The website of the CDC focused on the immunization schedule for adults is a quality resource that can be found at https://www.cdc.gov/vaccines/schedules/easy-to-read/adult.html

EXERCISE 4: CONDUCTING CRITICAL APPRAISALS TO BUILD AN EVIDENCE-BASED PRACTICE

Problem and Purpose

Hallas, Koslap-Petraco, and Fletcher (2017) Study

1. a. Significance of the problem: "During the toddler years, temper tantrums and impulsive behaviors are the norm. These behaviors can frustrate even the most experienced mothers. This frustration is evident in the 2014 national data that show the youngest children are the most vulnerable: 27% of the reported victims of child abuse and neglect are under the age of three (Center for Disease Control and Prevention [CDC] Injury Prevention and Control Division of Violence Prevention, 2016). Children's Bureau An Office of the Administration for Children and Families (2014) (https://www.childwelfare.gov/pubPDFs/fatality.pdf) reported that an estimated 1580 children died from child abuse and neglect, representing a rate of four children dying every day in the U.S. from abuse and neglect. Children under the age of three accounted for 70.7% of these fatalities: 40.1% were infants and 33.6% were between one and three years old" (Hallas et al., 2017, p. 33).

    b. Background of the problem: "Toddler behaviors viewed as problematic by mothers have been linked to maternal negative behaviors and stress (Calkins, 2002). Adverse toddler behaviors have been identified as a precursor to low maternal self-esteem and a lack of maternal confidence... Walker and Sprague (2000) concluded that once social-emotional problems are established in a young child, it is difficult to alter their behavior, as the children are highly resistant to change. Other researchers have confirmed that untreated social-emotional problems become chronic problems as the child continues to age" (Hallas et al., 2017, pp. 33–34).

    c. Problem statement: "Thus, an urgency to implement strategies to improve mother–toddler interactions, the social-emotional development of toddlers, and potentially reduce the potential for harm to toddlers was the rationale for the study design" (Hallas et al., 2017, p. 34).

2. Study purpose: "The focus of this study was to evaluate the effectiveness of a pediatric primary care office-based parenting skills intervention to improve 1) maternal confidence in caring for a toddler and 2) the social-emotional development of toddlers" (Hallas et al., 2017, p. 34).

3. Yes, the problem and purpose are significant because a large number of toddlers are abused and neglected and several die as a result. The toddler stage is difficult for mothers to manage, and they need support to prevent the development of social-emotional problems in their toddlers that could become chronic if not treated. The maternal problems in caring for toddlers stress the need for strategies to improve their parenting skills (see the Problem discussion in Question 1). The research purpose clearly addresses the identified problem.

4. Yes, the variables, population, and setting were identified in the study purpose.

    a. This randomized controlled trial (RCT) focuses on determining the effectiveness of an intervention on selected outcomes. The independent variable was a videotape (DVD) of parenting skills intervention. The dependent variables were social-emotional development of the toddlers and maternal confidence for mothers raising toddlers.

    b. Population: Mothers and toddlers dyads or pairs

    c. Settings: Pediatric primary care offices

5. The problem and purpose are feasible because (a) Hallas, Koslap-Petraco, and Fletcher had the research, educational, and clinical expertise to conduct this study, as discussed in Chapter 1 of this study guide; (b) the study was funded by the New York University Research Fund; (c) adequate study participants were available because the population included mothers of toddlers in five pediatric primary care offices; (d) clinic personnel were supportive of the study; (e) arrangements were made for implementing the intervention and collecting data on the study outcomes in appropriate places; and (f) the study was ethical and protected the rights of the study participants.

Erikson and Davies (2017) Study

1. a. Significance of the problem: "Pediatric palliative care (PPC) is an approach to care that emphasizes providing comprehensive care to children with life-threatening conditions and their families (American Academy of Pediatrics [AAP], 2013). In Western nations, children in need of PPC are diagnosed with life-threatening illnesses, such as congenital disorders, progressive chronic conditions, or acute, serious illnesses that may place a child at risk for premature death… Consequently, registered nurses in these settings must attend not only to children's physical and medical needs, but also to

their and their families' emotional, psychosocial, and spiritual needs" (Erikson & Davies, 2017, p. 42).

b. Background of the problem: "Families of seriously ill children strongly desire and deeply appreciate genuine emotional support and empathic communication from healthcare providers, especially at the end of life and after their child's death (Contro, Larson, Scofield, Sourkes, & Cohen, 2002; Davies, Larson, Contro, & Cabrera, 2011…)… Nurses caring for children at the end of life experience sadness and grief, but offering emotional support to families is an essential aspect of their practice from which they derive meaning and work satisfaction (Bloomer, O'Connor, Copnell, & Endacott, 2015…)" (Erikson & Davies, 2017, p. 42).

c. Problem statement: "It is to be expected that nurses who practice in these emotionally charged situations confront issues related to professional boundaries but little is known about how nurses manage professional and personal boundaries within the context of PPC" (Erikson & Davies, 2017, pp. 42–43).

2. a. "Purpose: To explore how nurses manage personal and professional boundaries in caring for seriously ill children and their families" (Erikson & Davies, 2017, p. 42). "The purpose of this paper is to describe how pediatric nurses defined boundaries and present a theoretical conceptualization of an identified process for managing boundaries, entitled maintaining integrity" (Erikson & Davies, 2017, p. 43).

b. Erikson and Davies (2017) provided two different purpose statements that need to be combined to provide a clear, complete focus for this grounded theory study.

c. The purpose of this study was to describe how pediatric nurses define their personal and professional boundaries and to present a theoretical conceptualization of an identified process for managing boundaries, entitled maintaining integrity.

3. Yes, the problem and purpose are significant because children with life-threatening illnesses and their families need comprehensive care that might best be provided through PPC. Nurses caring for these children and their families experience many emotions that require support, and they need direction in navigating the boundaries of PPC.

4. Erikson and Davies identified the study concepts and population but not the setting.

a. The research concepts studied with grounded theory included: Personal and professional

boundaries within the context of PPC and the process for managing these boundaries.

b. Population for the study was nurses providing PPC to seriously ill children and their families.

c. The setting for this study was not provided in the purpose. However, the two settings used were addressed in the design and methods section as a freestanding palliative care center and a tertiary-care children's hospital.

5. The problem and purpose of this study were feasible because: (a) the researchers had educational, clinical, and research expertise to conduct this study as detailed in Chapter 1 of this study guide; (b) the study was supported by the Betty Irene Moore Pre-doctoral Fellowship at the University of California, San Francisco; (c) an adequate number of RNs was available for this qualitative study from the PPC center and children's hospital; (d) data were collected through interviews conducted in private and convenient places within these two settings; and (e) the study methods appeared ethical with approval to conduct the study obtained from the university and clinical agencies institutional review boards.

Wendler, Smith, Ellenburg, Gill, Anderson, and Spiegel-Thayer (2017) Study

1. a. Significance of the problem: "Long separations are a characteristic of the day of surgery, keeping patients and their family members waiting and apart. At a time of high vulnerability, these separations can cause anxiety and worry… Less than 20% of American postanesthesia care units (PACUs) allow family visitation in the first hour after surgery despite strong advocacy by researchers and the American Society of PeriAnesthesia Nurses for patient/family visits" (Wendler et al., 2017, p. 45).

b. Background of the problem: "Restricting visitation during the recovery phase is in conflict with the needs of family members who, in one study, identified the need to visit a family member soon after surgery as one of their top two needs.[4] Indeed, families 'have consistently indicated strong support for visitation… [because of their need to know] that their loved one is safe and comfortable'"[1] (Wendler et al., 2017, p. 45).

c. Problem statement: "Despite the evidence that supports PACU visitation, including the safety and efficacy of such visits, family visits were not routine at this 500-bed Magnet-designated facility… Anecdotally, the nursing staff wondered: Were phase 1 visits safe for the patient and family member? And would these visits reduce anxiety and increase satisfaction with care?" (Wendler et al., 2017, pp. 45–46).

2. "The purpose of this study was to identify the outcomes and experiences of patients and family members who engaged in a 5- to 10-minute supervised family visit during phase I postanesthesia recovery" (Wendler et al., 2017, p. 45). "The purpose of this study was to discover and describe the experiences of total joint replacement patients and their family members who participated in a brief family visit during phase 1 [postanesthesia] recovery" (Wendler et al., 2017, p. 46). No, the researchers stated the study purpose in slightly different words three places on pages 45–46. Two of these purpose statements are included in this answer. Restating the study purpose using different words can be confusing to the reader.

3. Yes, the problem is significant since more than 80% of the PACUs do not allow family visitation in the first hour after surgery. Research evidence supports family visitation in the PACUs to promote safe, quality recovery for the patient and family. Thus, this descriptive, mixed methods study was conducted to examine the outcomes and experience of patients and family members following a supervised visit in the PACU. The purpose builds upon the problem statement and clearly indicates the focus of the study.

4. Examining the two purpose statements presented for Question 2, the research concepts, populations, and setting can be identified.
   a. The research concepts are outcomes and experiences of patients and family members who engaged in a 5- to 10-minute family visit intervention. This mixed methods study was not focused on testing the effectiveness of an intervention but on describing the outcomes and experiences of patients and family members following a visitation.
   b. The populations are total joint replacement patients and their family members.
   c. The setting was the PACU.

5. The problem and purpose of this study were feasible because (a) the study was funded by the Society of PeriAnesthesia Nurses and Memorial Medical Center Foundation in Illinois, indicating strong professional support for the research; (b) the researchers have the educational, clinical, and research expertise to conduct this study, as was discussed in Chapter 1 of this study guide; (c) the PACU in a 500-bed Magnet-designated hospital included an adequate pool of potential study participants ($n = 62$ patient and family member dyads or pairs); (d) the hospital

provided the necessary equipment and appropriate setting for the study; and (e) the study seemed ethical with potential benefits and limited risks, institutional approval, and participants' informed consent.

Objectives, Questions, and Hypotheses
Hallas et al. (2017) Study

1. Hallas et al. (2017, p. 34) stated the following hypotheses to direct their RCT: "1. There will be a greater increase in the social-emotional development of toddlers as measured by the Brigance Toddler Screen for toddlers whose mothers receive the treatment intervention (treatment group) in a pediatric primary care office-based practice as compared to toddlers in the control group whose mothers receive the standard office-based care. 2. There will be a greater increase in maternal confidence for mothers who receive the parenting skills intervention (treatment group) in a pediatric primary care office-based practice as measured by the Toddler Care Questionnaire (TCQ) compared to mothers in the control group who receive the standard office-based care."

2. Yes, these hypotheses are appropriate for a RCT, which is an experimental quantitative study. This study was focused on examining the effects of a parenting skills intervention on outcomes for the toddler and mother. These hypotheses clearly directed the development of the design, the data analyses, and interpretation of study findings. The first hypothesis predicts the outcome of increased social-emotional development of the toddlers and the second hypothesis predicts increased maternal confidence. These hypotheses would have been stronger and more concise if the measurement methods were deleted.

Erikson and Davies (2017) Study

1. This grounded theory qualitative study did not include objectives or questions. The study purpose guided the conduct of this study.
2. The purpose did include different foci, such as defining professional and personal boundaries and conceptualizing the process for managing the boundaries. Research questions or objectives might have helped organize and clarified the results and discussion sections of this research report.

Wendler et al. (2017) Study

1. Wendler et al. (2017, p. 46) stated the following research questions to guide their study: "1. What is the description of phase 1 family visit related to

patients' state anxiety, mean blood pressure, and heart rate (HR) over time and satisfaction with the visit? 2. What is the description of phase 1 family visit related to *family members'* state anxiety and satisfaction with the visit? 3. What is the description of what it is like for both patients and family members who experience phase 1 family visit in the PACU?"

2. Yes, the research questions provide clear direction for the data collection, presentation of results, and the discussion of findings for this mixed methods study. The first two questions direct the descriptive quantitative part of the study, and the third question is addressed by the exploratory-descriptive qualitative part of the study.

Study Variables and Concepts
Hallas et al. (2017) Study

1. The key study variables are identified in the study hypotheses:

Variable	Type of variable
DVD parenting skills	Independent variable
Social-emotional development of toddlers	Dependent variable
Maternal confidence	Dependent variable

2. a. Conceptual definition of DVD parenting skills intervention: The two DVD interventions were "designed by the PI [principle investigator] and Co-I, were based on Watson's caring theoretical framework, specifically the helping–trusting relationship (Watson, 1997, 2003)… A helping and trusting relationship evolves in caring moments when the mother embraces the toddler in times of opposing emotions such as love/anger, happiness/frustration, and is accepting of both the positive and negative feelings expressed by the toddler" (Hallas et al., 2017, p. 34).

   b. Operational definition of DVD parenting skills intervention: "Two-treatment intervention DVDs were designed: One for teenage mothers and one for all other mothers. The only difference between the teenage mother intervention DVD and the treatment intervention DVD for all other mothers was an additional one-minute discussion on being a teenage mother. Teenage development in comparison to toddler development was discussed" (Hallas et al., 2017, p. 35). The contents of the DVDs are presented in Table 1 of the research report.

3. Yes, the conceptual and operational definitions for the DVD parenting skills intervention are clearly

and concisely expressed in this study. The conceptual definition was expressed in the study framework and has a strong link to the operational definition in the methods section. The definitions are easy for the readers to identify and understand.

4. The sample characteristics for this study are presented in Tables 5 and 6 of this study. The demographic variables included: race/ethnicity, help from babysitter, toddler in day care, other children in the home, mother's work status, mother's age in years, and baby's age in months.

Wendler et al. (2017) Study

1. Study variables and concepts

Variable or concept	Type of variable or concept
Patients' state anxiety	Research variable
Patients' blood pressure (BP)	Research variable
Patients' heart rate (HR)	Research variable
Patients' satisfaction with the visit	Research variable
Family members' state anxiety	Research variable
Family members' satisfaction with visit	Research variable
Patients' experiences with the visit	Research concept
Family members' experiences with the visit	Research concept

2. a. Conceptual definition of patients' state anxiety: "The theoretical underpinning of this study is Roy's adaptation model. This theory posits that the patient is a biopsychosocial being constantly in interaction with the environment. Stress is encountered in everyday life and extraordinary circumstances, and the human being responds to these stimuli in complex ways… Reducing the stress response of both the patient and the family member, here expressed as state anxiety…" (Wendler et al., 2017, p. 47).

   b. Operational definition of patients' state anxiety: This variable was measured with the Spielberger State-Trait Anxiety Inventory (STAI).

3. Yes, the researchers provided very clear and appropriate conceptual and operational definitions for the variable patients' state anxiety. The conceptual definition is clearly linked to the study framework, Roy's adaptation model. The conceptual definition provides

a basis for the operational definition. The STAI has strong validity and reliability and has been used frequently in nursing research for several decades.

4. The demographic variables included in this study were age, race, and gender for both the patients and family members. The sample characteristics are presented in Table 1 of this study.

CHAPTER 6—UNDERSTANDING AND CRITICALLY APPRAISING THE LITERATURE REVIEW

EXERCISE 1: TERMS AND DEFINITIONS

1. m
2. d
3. l
4. n
5. h
6. i
7. c
8. a
9. k
10. j
11. b
12. o
13. f
14. e
15. g

EXERCISE 2: LINKING IDEAS

Examples of Main Ideas from the Chapter

1. (1) relevant; (2) critically appraising; (3) synthesizing
2. known, not known
3. theoretical, scientific or empirical
4. five
5. quantitative
6. ethnographic
7. purpose
8. encyclopedia
9. valid, appropriate, current
10. summary table or conceptual map

Theoretical and Empirical Sources

1. T
2. E
3. E
4. T
5. T
6. E
7. E

8. E
9. T
10. E

Primary and Secondary Sources

1. S
2. P
3. P
4. P
5. P
6. P
7. S
8. S
9. P
10. P

EXERCISE 3: WEB-BASED INFORMATION AND RESOURCES

1. a. https://www.ninr.nih.gov/
   b. Located directly at https://www.ninr.nih.gov/sites/www.ninr.nih.gov/files/10-landmark-nursing-research-studies.pdf or by selecting the *Changing Practice, Changing Lives: 10 Landmark Nursing Research Studies* document from The National Institute of Nursing Research (NINR) publications page at https://www.ninr.nih.gov/newsandinformation/publications
   c. Answer will be one of the following:
   Aiken, L. H., Clarke, S. P., Sloane, D. M., Sochalski, J., & Silber, J. H. (2002) Hospital nurse staffing and patient mortality, nurse burnout, and job dissatisfaction. *Journal of the American Medical Association, 288*(16), 1987–1993.
   Bergstrom, N., Braden, B., Kemp, M., Champagne, M., & Ruby, E. (1996). Multisite study of incidence of pressure ulcers and the relationship between risk level, demographic characteristics, diagnoses, and prescription of preventive interventions. *Journal of the American Geriatrics Society, 44(*1), 22–30.
   Grey, M., Davidson, M., Boland, E. A., & Tamborlane, W. V. (2001). Clinical and psychosocial factors associated with achievement of treatment goals in adolescents with diabetes mellitus. *Journal of Adolescent Health, 28*(5), 377–385.
   Harrell, J. S., McMurray, R. G., Bangdiwala, S. I., Frauman, A. C., Gansky, S. A., & Bradley C. B. (1996). Effects of a school-based intervention to reduce cardiovascular disease risk factors in elementary-school children: The Cardiovascular Health in Children

(CHIC) Study. *The Journal of Pediatrics, 128* (6), 797–805.

Hill, M. N., Han, H., Dennison, C. R., Kim, M. T., Roary, M. C., Blumenthal, R. S. et al., (2003). Hypertension care and control in underserved urban African American men: Behavioral and physiologic outcomes at 36 months. *American Journal of Hypertension, 16*(11)*,* 906–913.

Jemmott, J. B., Jemmott, L. S., & Fong, G. T. (1998) Abstinence and safer sex HIV risk reduction interventions for African American adolescents: A randomized controlled trial. *Journal of the American Medical Association, 279*(19), 1529–1536.

Gear, R. W., Miaskowski, C., Gordon, N. C., Paul, S. M., Heller, P. H., & Levine, J. D. (1999). The kappa opioid nalbuphine produces gender- and dose-dependent analgesia and antianalgesia in patients with postoperative pain. *Pain, 83*(2), 339–345.

Lorig, K., Gonzalez, V. M., & Ritter, P. (1999). Community-based Spanish language arthritis education program: A randomized trial. *Medical Care, 37*(9), 957–963.

Naylor, M. D., Brooten, D. A., Campbell, R. L., Maislin, G., McCauley, K. M., & Schwartz, J. S. (2004). Transitional care of older adults hospitalized with heart failure: A randomized, controlled trial. *Journal of the American Geriatrics Society, 52*(5), 675–684.

Kitzman H., Olds, D. L., Henderson, C. R., Hanks, C., Cole, R., Tatelbaum, R. et al., (1997). Effect of prenatal and infancy home visitation by nurses on pregnancy outcomes, childhood injuries, and repeated childbearing: A randomized controlled trial. *Journal of the American Medical Association, 278*(8), 644–652.

2. Branson, S. M., Boss, L., Padhye, N. S., Trötscher, T., & Ward, A. (2017). Effects of animal assisted activities on biobehavioral stress responses in hospitalized children: A randomized controlled study. *Journal of Pediatric Nursing, 36*, 84–91.
   a. Randomized controlled trial or study
   b. Sample size $N = 48$
3. Endnote or RefWorks

EXERCISE 4: CONDUCTING CRITICAL APPRAISALS TO BUILD AN EVIDENCE-BASED PRACTICE

1. a. journal title
   b. year of publication
   c. volume number
   d. page numbers
   e. issue number
   f. Donna Hallas

g. Social-emotional development of toddlers: Randomized controlled trial of an office-based intervention.

2. Erikson, A., & Davies, B. (2017). Maintaining integrity: How nurses navigate boundaries in pediatric palliative care. *Journal of Pediatric Nursing, 35*, 42–49.

3. a. The *Journal of PeriAnesthesia Nursing* website is located at http://www.jopan.org/
   b. Yes, the *Journal of PeriAnesthesia Nursing* is peer reviewed. Confirmation can be found on the *Journal of PeriAnesthesia Nursing* homepage http://www.jopan.org/ under "About *Journal of PeriAnesthesia Nursing*"

4. a. toddler, social-emotional development, and maternal confidence
   b. pediatric palliative care, nursing, nurses, boundaries, and grounded theory
   c. PACU, family visitation, and postanesthesia recovery

5. Introduction at the beginning of the study and the Background section of the Hallas et al. (2017, pp. 42–43) study include the review of literature

6. Five references

7. a. Yes. For example, *Journal of Pediatric Nursing, Journal of Pediatric Oncology Nursing, and Pediatric Nursing* are peer-reviewed journals.
   b. Yes. For example, Bloomer et al. (2015) and Price et al. (2011) are primary sources because they are research reports written by researchers who conducted the studies.
   c. No, the authors do not explicitly justify the references that are not peer-reviewed, primary sources but they are appropriate for use in the literature review. For example, Charmaz (2014) is a book used for grounded theory methodology.
   d. Yes, previous studies are described. Previous theory is not described but appropriate to the grounded theory methodology, theory development is discussed.

8. a. Within 10 years $36/48 = 0.75 \times 100 = 75\%$; Within 5 years $25/48 = 0.52 \times 100 = 52\%$ Despite using older literature, the literature review provided adequate background to logically support the purpose of the study. Grounded theory studies are typically conducted in areas with minimal literature and may therefore have a greater number of older sources.
   b. Chosen older studies such as Contro et al. (2002) and Rashotte et al. (1997) are widely cited by other researchers, which is an indication that they are probably seminal or landmark studies. Replication studies are reproductions and repetitions of a study, which

are unlikely references for a grounded theory study that seeks to generate new knowledge in an area with limited research.

c. No, Charmaz (2014), the book used as a grounded theory methodology reference, and Polit and Beck (2016), the book used as an approach for establishing trustworthiness in qualitative research, were current references.

9. a. Yes, the content is directly related to the study concepts such as boundaries and palliative care.

b. Yes, most sources were from the discipline of nursing and others were from medicine, which is appropriate for the study. Quantitative and qualitative studies were included.

10. a. No, the quality of the included studies were not addressed; therefore, the studies were not critically appraised.

b. Yes, studies were well synthesized. Studies with similar findings were summarized together. Presented findings related to pediatric palliative care and boundaries were connected together in a logical flow.

c. Yes, a clear concise summary of what is known about pediatric palliative care, emotional impact on nurses, and boundaries was presented. Erikson and Davies (2017, p. 43) provided a summary sentence of what is known: "Caring for seriously ill children who may die affects pediatric nurses on a personal level." Erikson and Davies (2017, p. 43) identified the gap in the literature by stating "little was known about how pediatric nurses manage professional and personal boundaries."

d. Yes, Erikson and Davies (2017, p. 43) clearly linked the gap in the literature (presented in answer 10b) to the study purpose: "Understanding how nurses manage professional boundaries must also include examining their personal boundaries, thus the overall aim of our study was to explore how nurses perceived and managed professional and personal boundaries." The gap is also linked to the choice of grounded theory as a methodology.

CHAPTER 7 — UNDERSTANDING THEORY AND RESEARCH FRAMEWORKS

EXERCISE 1: TERMS AND DEFINITIONS

1. j
2. h
3. e
4. b
5. c
6. i

7. a
8. f
9. g
10. k
11. d

Types of Theories

1. e
2. a
3. b
4. f
5. d
6. c

EXERCISE 2: LINKING IDEAS

Key Theoretical Ideas

1. statements, propositions, relationships among concepts
2. variable
3. propositions or relational statements
4. hypotheses
5. Conceptual definitions are abstract, comprehensive definitions based on theory. Operational definitions are narrower and indicate how the variable will be measured, implemented, or observed in the specific study.
6. Grand nursing theories are abstract conceptual models that describe nursing. Middle range theories are less abstract and focus on a specific phenomenon or situation in practice. The example of a grand nursing theory may be any of the theories listed in Table 7.3 or another grand theory identified by searching the Internet. The example of a middle range theory may be any of the theories listed in Table 7.4 or another middle range nursing theory identified by searching the Internet.
7. Orem
8. nursing intellectual capital
9. Mishel's Theory of Uncertainty for Acute and Chronic Illness

Levels of Abstraction

Construct (*highest*)
Concept
Variable
Operational definition (*lowest*)

Elements of Theory

1. physical health, psychological health, quality of life
2. relationships between the concepts, also called propositions
3. research framework

Examples of Frameworks

1. g
2. a
3. h
4. d
5. b
6. e
7. c
8. f

Example of Grand Theory Used in a Study

1. 64 persons who had had an acute myocardial infarction and were in inpatient rehabilitation
2. King's Goal Attainment Theory
3. b. Development of the intervention, a goal-oriented education program

EXERCISE 3: WEB-BASED INFORMATION AND RESOURCES

1. a. 1) relief, 2) ease, and 3) transcendence
   b. http://currentnursing.com/nursing_theory/ comfort_theory_Kathy_Kolcaba.html (URL may vary)
2. a. Will depend on which grand theory student selects and the information found:
      Adaptation Model (Roy & Andrews, 2008) http:// currentnursing.com/nursing_theory/application _Roy's_adaptation_model.html
      Self-Care Deficit Theory of Nursing (Orem, 2001) http://currentnursing.com/nursing_theory/ application_self_care_deficit_theory.html
      Science of Unitary Human Beings (Rogers, 1970) http://currentnursing.com/nursing_theory/ unitary_human_beings.html
      Theory of Goal Attainment (King, 1992) http://currentnursing.com/nursing_theory/ application_goal_attainment_theory.html
   b. Adaptation Model–focal, contextual, and residual stimuli; cognator subsystem, regulator subsystem, modes of adaptation: physiological needs, self-concept, role function, interdependence.
      Self-Care Deficit Theory–nursing systems (wholly compensatory, partially compensatory, and supportive-educative systems), self care deficit, therapeutic self care, health deviation self care.
      Science of Unitary Human Beings–energy field, openness, pattern, pan-dimensionality,
      Theory of Goal Attainment-personal, interpersonal, and social systems, transaction, communication, mutually-agreed-upon goals.

EXERCISE 4: CONDUCTING CRITICAL APPRAISALS TO BUILD AN EVIDENCE-BASED PRACTICE

Hallas, Koslap-Petraco, & Fletcher (2017)

1. Watson
2. Helping, trusting relationship
3. a. parental stress and psychological health
   b. Hypothesis 1. "There will be a greater increase in the social-emotional development of toddlers as measured by the Brigance Toddler Screen for toddlers whose mothers receive the treatment intervention (treatment group) in a pediatric primary care office-based practice as compared to toddlers in the control group whose mothers receive the standard office-based care" (p. 34).

Wendler, Smith, Ellenburg, Gill, Anderson, and Spiegel-Thayer (2017)

4. Roy's adaptation model
5. The answers to the question are provided in the table below.

Phrases From the Article	Related Concept of the Theory	Conceptual Definition
Overall surgical experience/ event	Focal stimuli	The primary threat to adaptation confronting the person right now.
Past healthcare experiences and prior coping for the family as a whole	Residual stimuli	Previous experiences that affect the current situation but how they affect the situation is unclear.
Enforcement of separation of patient from family members during phase 1 recovery	Contextual stimuli	Other stimuli in the environment that are affecting the situation.
Family visit to mitigate incomplete coping	Cognitive-emotive and regulator subsystems	Adaptive responses that are mental or emotional, such as learning, making a judgment, or processing information. Adaptive responses that are automatic through neural, chemical, or endocrine channels.

6. State anxiety
7. Wendler et al. (2017) identified Roy's adaptation model as the theoretical underpinning of the study. The researchers provided conceptual definitions for the patient as "a biopsychosocial being constantly in interaction with the environment" (p. 47), stress as "everyday life and extraordinary circumstances" to which the "human being responds to… in complex ways" (p. 47), and the goal of nursing care as supporting the "successful coping of the patient as she or he becomes integrated and whole" (p. 47). However, these concepts were not the concepts that were measured (operationalized) for the study. As shown in the table above, the researchers did link the model's concepts of focal stimuli, residual stimuli, contextual stimuli, and cognitive-emotive and regulator subsystems to the experience being studied and the environment of the PACU. The researchers explained the theoretical basis for the nursing intervention and identified reducing stress as the goal of the intervention, which was operationalized as state anxiety. The goal of the intervention was the only concept for which a conceptual definition was implied and an operational definition found (score on the Spielberger State-Trait Anxiety Inventory). For the intervention, the conceptual and operational definitions were consistent with each other. The relationships being studied were the effect of the family visit on the patient's state anxiety, vital signs, and satisfaction with the visit and on the family member's state anxiety and satisfaction with the visit. The relationships were identified in the first and second research questions. In the Discussion section of the article, Wendler et al. (2017) linked the study findings back to the theory by stating "Roy's adaptation model would predict that the family visit would modulate the stress of waiting after surgery through coping, and this, in fact, was the result" (p. 53). Although conceptual definitions for all the variables were not provided, the study was a strong example of using a grand theory to guide an intervention study.

CHAPTER 8—CLARIFYING QUANTITATIVE RESEARCH DESIGNS

EXERCISE 1: TERMS AND DEFINITIONS

Understanding Common Design Terms

1. n
2. a
3. l
4. e
5. c
6. d
7. i
8. j
9. f
10. k
11. h
12. g
13. m
14. b

Design Validity Terms

1. b
2. e
3. h
4. f
5. a
6. i
7. c
8. j
9. g
10. d

EXERCISE 2: LINKING IDEAS

1. effects or outcomes
2. treatment, intervention, or independent variable
3. cause and effect, causality, or the effect of an intervention on a study outcome
4. control
5. descriptive correlational design
6. cause; effect or outcome; cause
7. design validity
8. predictive correlational
9. treatment, intervention, or experimental group; control or comparison group
10. intervention fidelity
11. control
12. comparative descriptive
13. model testing
14. You might have listed any three of the following elements:
    a. The study includes a treatment or intervention.
    b. The experimental or treatment group receives the study intervention.
    c. The intervention is manipulated by the researchers to create an outcome or effect.
    d. The study usually includes a control or comparison group.
    e. The extraneous variables are controlled as much as possible to reduce their influence on study findings.
    f. The study participants should be randomly assigned to either the intervention or control group.
    g. The study is strengthened if the study participants are randomly selected for the study.
15. large samples

Determining Types of Design Validity in Studies

1. c
2. d
3. a
4. b
5. a
6. c
7. b
8. d
9. a
10. b

Identifying a Design Model

1. A descriptive correlational design model is presented in Figure 8.6 of your textbook *Understanding Nursing Research*, 7th edition.

2. Quasi-experimental pretest and post-test design with comparison group model is presented in Figure 8.10 of your textbook *Understanding Nursing Research*, 7th edition.

Control and Designs for Nursing Studies

1. **Quasi-experimental post-test-only design with comparison group**—this study examined the effect of an animated program on DVD on children's pain during IV insertion. The DVD controlled the content and the implementation of the intervention to ensure intervention fidelity. The FACES rating scale is a quality method for measuring acute pain in children. The age of the children was controlled, as was the setting for the study. The children were obtained by a sample of convenience and were not randomly assigned to groups, but the groups were equal in number. There is a possible threat to internal design validity since the children were placed in a group based on their hospital unit and these units might have been different in some way.

2. **Correlational study**—the relationships among the variables of hours of sleep, stress level, anxiety level, and depression were measured in first-time mothers. Limiting the sample to first-time mothers in the first month following the birth of their child was a way of controlling extraneous variables. The measurement methods in this study are unknown but need to be reliable and valid. Correlational studies have less control than quasi-experimental studies so the population might be studied without manipulation in a natural setting.

3. **Predictive correlational design**—the independent variables perception of self-esteem, depression level, age, and educational level were used to predict the dependent variable self-care abilities of women being treated for lung cancer. This correlation study identified a specific population and the variables should be measured with reliable and valid instruments. Determining the sample size using power analysis strengthens the study's statistical conclusion validity.

4. **Comparative descriptive design**—the study's purpose focused on describing and examining the differences between males' and females' health promotion behaviors. The study population was limited to people with type 2 diabetes in primary care clinics. Conducting a power analysis to determine the sample size for the study would have strengthened the statistical conclusion validity. The health promotion behaviors would need to be measured with a quality scale.

5. **Quasi-experimental pretest and post-test design with comparison group**—examining the effects of vitamins on infant weight gain. Data collection was controlled with the pretest being done prior to implementing the vitamin intervention and the post-test was conducted at 8 months of age. The intervention of vitamins was controlled by using a detailed protocol for implementation. The sample was one of convenience obtained from three pediatricians' offices; however, the participants were randomly assigned to the intervention and comparison groups. The adequacy of the sample size needs to be determined with power analysis.

6. **Randomized controlled trial (RCT)**—testing the effectiveness of a new hypertensive medication. The study has a large sample size with random assignment to the comparison and intervention groups. The study was conducted in multiple sites and two different geographical areas. In addition, the medication intervention was manipulated in a controlled way to ensure the right participants got the medication and that the medication was delivered accurately at the right time, right dose, and right route. Measurement of blood pressure (BP) was controlled to ensure precise and accurate readings.

EXERCISE 3: WEB-BASED INFORMATION AND RESOURCES

1. CONsolidated Standards for Reporting Trials (CONSORT).
   The CONSORT website is: http://www.consort-statement.org

2. a. Sethares and Asselin (2017, p. 192) reported a "one-group mixed method pre-test/post-test design" was implemented in their study. The quantitative part of the design was a one-group quasi-experimental design and the qualitative aspect appeared to be exploratory descriptive.
   b. "Self-care behaviors were measured using the 22 item revised Self-Care of Heart Failure Index" (Sethares & Asselin, 2017, p. 194).

EXERCISE 4: CONDUCTING CRITICAL APPRAISALS TO BUILD AN EVIDENCE-BASED PRACTICE

Hallas, Koslap-Petraco and Fletcher (2017) Study

1. The Hallas et al. (2017, p. 33, p. 35) study included a "prospective, double blind, randomized controlled trial [RCT] using a pretest/post-test experimental design."

2. Yes, the study design is clearly identified in the abstract and the methods section of the research report (see the answer to Question 1). The title also indicated that a RCT was conducted. RCT is an experimental design and the authors specified the type of experimental design.

3. Yes, the intervention implemented in this study was a videotaped (DVD) of parenting skills. Two intervention DVDs were designed for the study: "one for teenage mothers and one for all other mothers. The only difference between the teenage mother intervention DVD and the treatment intervention DVD for all other mothers was an additional one-minute discussion on being a teenage mother" (Hallas et al., 2017, p. 35).

4. Yes, the study included a control group that received a standardized DVD on toddler nutrition. The DVDs used for the control group were wrapped the same as the intervention DVDs so the mothers, RNs, and research assistants (RAs) were blinded to the group assignment (either the treatment or control group).

5. The design validity strengths in the Hallas et al. (2017) study are identified as follows. You might have selected any four of the following strengths. If you identify additional validity strengths, ask your faculty about them for clarification.
   a. **Construct validity:** The variables were clearly conceptually defined "based on Watson's Caring theoretical framework, specifically the helping trusting relationship" (Hallas et al., 2017, p. 34).
   b. **Construct validity:** The Toddler Care Questionnaire (TCQ) was developed in 1988 and has been used in several previous studies. The items on TCQ were included in the study and were focused on measuring maternal confidence. The Brigance Toddler Screen was developed in 2002 and has been used in previous studies, adding to the validity of the instrument. The items on the Brigance Toddler screen were focused on the social-emotional skills of toddlers.
   c. **Construct validity:** The mothers, RNs, and RAs were blinded to group assignment, which controlled the potential for bias.
   d. **Internal validity:** The mother and child dyads were randomized into either the intervention or control group. The randomization of participants to groups was accomplished by a biostatistician using a computer-generated list of random numbers.
   e. **Internal validity:** No evidence that a historical event affected the outcomes of the study.
   f. **External validity:** The interaction of selection and intervention were limited since the DVDs for the intervention and control group were in the same wrapper, blinding the mothers, RNs, and RAs to the type of DVD they were watching.
   g. **External validity:** There seemed to be no historical event that interacted with the intervention.
   h. **Statistical conclusion validity:** The TCQ and the Brigance Toddler Screen have strong documented reliability.
   i. **Statistical conclusion validity:** The intervention content was rigorously developed and included in Table 1 in the study. The content was consistently delivered using DVDs, supporting intervention fidelity.
   j. **Statistical conclusion validity:** The demographic variables for the treatment and control groups were not significantly different at the start of the study except for the mother's age (see Table 6), which decreases the potential influence of extraneous variables.

6. The threats to design validity in the Hallas et al. (2017) study are identified as follows. You might have selected any two of the following threats. If you identified different threats to design validity, ask your faculty about them.
   a. **Construct validity threat:** This study has mono-operation bias since the study variables were measured by only one instrument each. Maternal confidence was measured with the TCQ and the social-emotional development of the toddlers was measured by the Brigance Toddler Screen as indicated in the study hypotheses and the methods section.
   b. **Internal validity:** This study had fairly high participant attrition, since nine mothers did not complete the second visit resulting in 26 mother–toddler dyads in the treatment group and 25 mother–toddler dyads in the control group.
   c. **Statistical conclusion validity threat:** The power analysis indicated that each group should include 30 mother–toddler dyads. The attrition caused the study to have low statistical power (less than 30 in both the treatment and control groups), which might have contributed to selected nonsignificant findings. The sample size should be large enough to accommodate the attrition of mother–toddler dyads during the study.

d. **Internal validity threat:** Both the control and the treatment groups improved so there might have been a maturation affect that biased the study results. Both groups received a DVD educational program that might have affected both groups' scores on the study instruments.

e. **External validity threat:** The study took place in five pediatric primary healthcare offices and the researchers noted the participants from some of the sites were different than others based on the demographic information. This indicates a potential interaction of setting and intervention.

7. The following elements of the study were controlled:

a. The intervention content was rigorously controlled during development.

b. The intervention was consistently implemented using a DVD.

c. Control group received a standardized DVD, blinding mothers, RNs, and RAs to the group assignment.

d. A power analysis was conducted to identify the sample size needed for determining the effectiveness of the DVD intervention.

e. The assignment to groups was controlled through randomization by a statistician.

f. The TCQ and Brigance Toddler Screen demonstrated validity and reliability and the items of the two instruments were included in the study.

g. RAs were trained to ensure consistent data collection.

h. The data collection process was highly structured.

Wendler, Smith, Ellenburg, Gill, Anderson, and Spiegel-Thayer (2017) Study

1. The design of the Wendler et al. (2017, p. 45, 47) study "was a descriptive, single-group, mixed-methods study."

2. Yes, the design was clearly identified in the abstract and methods section of the research report. The specific design is identified in Question 1.

3. The quantitative part of the study design was comparative descriptive. The patients' state anxiety, blood pressure, and heart rate were described and compared before and after their family members' visit. The family members' state anxiety was described and also compared before and after their visit with the patient. The satisfaction scores for both the patients and family members were measured using the following question: "On a scale of 0-4, with zero meaning 'not at all satisfied'

and four meaning 'the most satisfied I can be,' how satisfied were you with your family visit?" (Wendler et al., 2017, p. 50). The satisfaction scores were analyzed only with descriptive statistics and were not compared across the two measurements.

4. The design validity strengths in the Wendler et al. (2017) study are identified as follows. You might have selected any three of the following strengths. If you identify additional validity strengths, ask your faculty about them for clarification.

a. **Construct validity:** The variables were clearly conceptually defined using Roy's Adaptation Model and these definitions were appropriately linked to the operational definitions.

b. **Construct validity:** Patient and family state anxiety levels were measured using the Spielberger State-Trait Anxiety Inventory (STAI), which has been used in many nursing studies over the years and reported to be valid. The STAI "has been developed for all ages, translated into several languages, and is written at the fourth-grade level" (Wendler et al., 2017, p. 50). The vital signs of mean arterial pressure (MAP) and heart rate (HR) were measured using the Dräger Infinity Delta monitor, which ensured the accuracy of these readings.

c. **Internal validity:** The researchers had no attrition during the study with the sample size being 62 patient/family member dyads throughout the study.

d. **Internal validity:** No evidence of a historical event affected the outcomes of the study.

e. **Statistical conclusion validity:** The study had an adequate sample size and power to detect differences for patients and family members. "Table 2 illustrates the patients' and family members' mean STAI before and after the visit, indicating a clinically and statistically significant reduction in state anxiety after the visit ($p < .001$)" (Wendler et al., 2017, p. 52).

f. **Statistical conclusion validity:** The STAI has reported reliability and the tool's reliability for this study was strong at 0.92. The MAP and HR were measured using the Dräger Infinity Delta monitor, which ensured the precision or reliability of these readings.

g. **Statistical conclusion validity:** The study was conducted in a postanesthesia care unit (PACU) in a "level 1 trauma, academically affiliated 500-bed Magnet hospital in the Midwest" (Wendler et al., 2017, p. 48). This is a single, controlled setting, which limits the influences of extraneous variables.

5. You might have selected any two of the following threats to design validity for the Wendler et al. (2017) study. If you identified additional threats to design validity, ask your faculty about them.

   a. **Construct validity threat:** This study has mono-operation bias since two of the study variables were measured by only one instrument each. State anxiety was measured by STAI and satisfaction with the visit was measured with a rating scale developed by the researchers.

   b. **Construct validity threat:** The satisfaction with the visit rating scale was a single item with ratings of 0 to 4 developed for this study with no evidence of validity or that it measured what it was supposed to in this study.

   c. **Internal validity:** Maturation might have occurred when the variables were measured before and after the visit, which could affect the study results.

   d. **Statistical conclusion validity threat:** The satisfaction with the visit rating scale was developed for this study, included only one item, and has undetermined reliability.

6. No. The focus of this mixed methods study was exploration of experiences and description and comparison of patients' and family members' anxiety and satisfaction after a family visit in the PACU. The focus is not on controlling of extraneous variables to determine the effect of an intervention on outcome variables.

CHAPTER 9—EXAMINING POPULATIONS AND SAMPLES IN RESEARCH

EXERCISE 1: TERMS AND DEFINITIONS
1. j
2. a
3. n
4. g
5. k
6. f
7. m
8. i
9. l
10. b
11. d
12. e
13. h
14. c
15. o

EXERCISE 2: LINKING IDEAS
1. elements
2. target population
3. sample, accessible population, and target population
4. You might identify any of the following:
   a. Compare the demographic characteristics of the sample with those of the target population determined from previous research.
   b. Compare mean sample values of study variables with the values of the target population determined from previous research.
   c. Identify the refusal rate in the study and identify the reasons potential subjects refused to participate. The lower the refusal rate and the more common the reasons for refusing to participate, the more representative the sample is of the target population.
   d. Evaluate the possibilities of systematic bias in the sample in terms of the setting, characteristics of the sample, and ranges of values on measured variables.
   e. Determine sample attrition rate and identify the reasons for the attrition or withdrawal of participants from the study. The lower the attrition rate and the more common or usual the reasons for attrition, the more representative the sample is of the target population.
5. the expected difference in values that occurs when different subjects from the same sample are examined
6. sampling frame
7. strategies or method(s) used to obtain a sample for a study
8. You might choose any of the following:
   a. Was the sampling plan adequately identified?
   b. Did the researcher successfully implement the sampling plan?
   c. Was the sampling plan effective in achieving representativeness of the target population?
   d. Were the subjects or participants selected from a sampling frame?
   e. Were the participants randomly selected?
9. homogeneous
10. heterogeneous
11. sampling criteria
12. sample characteristics
13. sample attrition
14. a. simple random sampling
    b. stratified random sampling
    c. cluster sampling
    d. systematic sampling
15. You might list any of the following:
    a. convenience sampling
    b. network sampling
    c. purposive sampling
    d. theoretical sampling
16. nonprobability
17. power analysis
18. differences or relationships
19. 0.8 or 80%
20. null hypothesis

21. You might list any of the following:
    a. effect size of a study
    b. type of study
    c. study design
    d. number of variables
    e. measurement sensitivity
    f. data analysis techniques
22. You might list any of the following:
    a. data saturation
    b. scope of the study
    c. nature of the topic
    d. quality of the information
    e. study design
23. inclusion and exclusion
24. Refusal number $= 250 - 208 = 42$. Refusal rate $=$ (42 refused $\div$ 250 subjects approached) $\times 100\% =$ $0.168 \times 100\% = 16.8\%$
25. Attrition rate $=$ (20 withdrew from the study $\div$ 150 sample size) $\times 100\% = 0.133 \times 100\% = 13.3\%$

Sampling Methods for Quantitative and Qualitative Studies

1. f	11. f
2. b	12. c
3. c	13. d
4. a	14. b
5. b	15. f
6. g	16. h
7. h	17. i
8. b	18. a
9. e	19. d
10. d	20. b

Determining Sample Size for Quantitative and Qualitative Studies

1. a	6. b
2. c	7. c
3. b	8. b
4. a	9. a
5. b	10. b

EXERCISE 3: WEB-BASED INFORMATION AND RESOURCES

1. You might have identified a variety of websites that discussed power analysis and a provide power analysis calculator. For example, G*Power provides an online program for understanding and conducting power analysis. Locate the free software at http://www.softpedia.com/get/Science-CAD/G-Power.shtml
   Some websites have useful information about research methodology; however, review the websites for quality of information. University websites usually provide more credible information than websites advertising products or services. Some websites will direct you to research articles and books that focus on power analysis and these could be excellent sources of information.
2. The English version of the World Health Organization (WHO) website is located at http://www.who.int/en/
3. Information on the WHO Multicentre Growth Reference Study (MGRS) http://www.who.int/childgrowth/mgrs/en/ and at http://www.who.int/childgrowth/mgrs/en/fnb_planning_p15_26.pdf?ua=1 the following reference can be obtained.
   Bhan, M. K., & Norum, K. R. (2004). The WHO multicentre growth reference study (MGRS): Rationale, planning, and implementation. Food and Nutrition Bulletin, 25(1 supplement 1).
4. international growth curves for infants and children
5. The sample size was approximately 8500 children.
6. Brazil, Ghana, India, Norway, Oman and the USA
7. Representativeness

EXERCISE 4: CONDUCTING CRITICAL APPRAISALS TO BUILD AN EVIDENCE-BASED PRACTICE

Hallas, Koslap-Petraco, and Fletcher (2017) Study

1. The study population was "mother–toddler dyads in which the mother was interacting with and raising the toddler" (p. 35).
2. Inclusion sample criteria were: "All mothers, who spoke English or Spanish, who were responsible for caring for a toddler who received their primary healthcare in one of the participating pediatric offices… All toddlers who were between the ages of 12 to 33 months at the start of the study and came for a primary health care visit with their mother met inclusion criteria as a mother–toddler dyad participant" (p. 35). Exclusion sample criteria: "All mothers of toddlers who could not speak or understand English or Spanish were excluded… Biological parents for children in foster care were excluded from this study, as they were not providing the day-to-day care for the toddler during the study period" (p. 35). No, the sampling criteria were not clearly stated since the exclusion criteria were mainly a repeat of the inclusion criteria. Inclusion and exclusion criteria should be distinctly different and identify potential study participants. Participants should be included if they meet the inclusion criteria and do not have the exclusion criteria.

3. The sample characteristics for the participants were presented in Table 6. A nonrandom sampling method conducted in the study reduced the sample's representativeness. However, the use of multiple geographically data collection sites (five pediatric primary healthcare offices) increased the representativeness of the sample. The researchers noted that "The offices and the clinic populations matched the general demographics of the boroughs and county, however our study sample differed in Queens and Brooklyn with a greater representation of Whites and Latinos than reported populations in these two boroughs" (p. 35). This sample seemed adequately representative of the target population based on the number of sites used, and the fact that potential study participants are limited in healthcare research so nonrandom sampling methods are often used.

4. Sample size was 60 mother–toddler dyads ($N = 60$) with $n = 29$ in the treatment group and $n = 31$ in the control group (see the abstract on page 33 or Table 5 on page 38).

5. The sample size was 60 mother–toddler dyads. A power analysis was conducted prior to data collection to determine an adequate sample size. "A prior power analysis was conducted for each outcome to ascertain the sample size necessary to attain a power of 0.80 with a type I error rate of 0.05… These analyses indicated a sample size of 30 mothers and toddlers for each group would provide sufficient power to detect the estimated effect" (p. 36). Researchers should have recruited more than 60 mother–toddler dyads to allow for adequate sample size after expected attrition. Researchers acknowledged "the small sample size that limited the statistical power" to be a limitation of the study (p. 39).

6. Attrition rate = (9 withdrew from the study ÷ 60 sample size) × 100% = 0.15 × 100% = 15% Table 5 compared those participants who completed the study versus those who dropped out.

7. Nonprobability sampling. Note that the randomization in this randomized controlled trial refers to the random assignment of participants into intervention and control groups and not random sampling to obtain participants.

8. Convenience sampling.

9. Hallas et al. (2017, p. 39) reported "The generalizability of this study is limited due to the small sample size that limited the statistical power of the study." The generalizability of the study findings is also decreased by the nonprobability sampling method.

10. Study setting: "Five pediatric primary healthcare offices participated as study sites and included offices in Brooklyn, Queens, Manhattan, and Suffolk County, New York" (p. 35). Researchers created a highly controlled setting by the use of controls in the form of a consistent DVD intervention that reduced possibility of intervention variation, group randomization and concealment of group allocation to participants and researchers (double blind).

Erikson and Davies (2013) Study

1. The population was pediatric registered nurses (RNs) who provided care to "seriously ill or dying children" (p. 44).

2. Sampling inclusion criteria: "participants were employed as RNs in one of the four study settings" (p. 43). No sample exclusion criteria were identified.

3. "The sample included 18 RNs (10 from the PPC center [pediatric palliative care center], 3 from the oncology unit, 3 from the ICN [intensive care nursery], and 2 from the PICU [pediatric intensive care unit])" (p. 43). Detailed sample characteristics were provided in Table 1. Under limitations, the researchers noted that "The majority of participants in the study were female, white and had a considerable number of years of nursing experience" (p. 48).

4. Sample size was $N = 18$ RNs.

5. The sample size of 18 was adequate for this qualitative, grounded theory study. The sample size is within a typical range for a qualitative study and more importantly, sample size was based on data saturation. The researcher noted, "Data saturation was achieved when new interviews added no new information" (p. 44).

6. nonprobability sampling

7. Erikson and Davies (2017) reported that convenience, purposeful, and network sampling methods were used to achieve their sample as indicated in the following quotes. "Using a constructivist grounded theory approach, a convenience sample of 18 registered nurses from four practice sites were interviewed" (p. 42). "Using purposeful sampling, RNs were recruited through approved flyers posted in each setting and through snowball sampling" (p. 43). The use of flyers is a method of convenience sampling. Snowball sampling is also called network sampling.

8. No, the study results cannot be generalized to the target population. Generalization is not the focus or goal of qualitative research.

9. Setting: "To enhance sampling variation, the principal investigator (PI) recruited registered nurses (RNs) from two sites: a freestanding pediatric palliative care center and an academic tertiary-care children's hospital, both situated in a large, metropolitan area in the Western United States… a mutually convenient time and place to meet for an

interview, most often in a private area at their workplace before or after their shift" (p. 43). This setting was appropriate to identify quality participants who could address the study purpose. The sites for the interviews were convenient and private to obtain the data needed to achieve data saturation.

Wendler, Smith, Ellenburg, Gill, Anderson, and Spiegel-Thayer (2017) Study

1. The population was "dyads, consisting of a patient and his or her selected family member" (Wendler et al., 2017, p. 48).
2. Inclusion criteria: "Patients 18 years and older underwent hip or knee replacement with spinal anesthesia. A family member was defined as any person (18 years and older) the patient designated" (Wendler et al., 2017, p. 48). Exclusion criteria: "if they did not have a designated family member present for the visit, if they did not want the visit, or if they were not willing to complete the consenting process" (p. 48).
3. Minimal characteristics of the homogenous sample were presented on Table 1. "Demographics revealed that patients and family members were similar to the general population of joint replacement patients at this hospital, comprising of primarily females (patient = 66% and family member = 69%) and Caucasian (patient = 95% and family member = 92%). The mean age of the patients was 62.9 (range, 30 to 87) and family members was 58.3 (range, 31 to 85)" (p. 52). This quote indicates that the sample was similar and thus probably representative of the target population.
4. Sample included 62 patients and their family member ($n = 62 + 62$) = 124 participants or 62 dyads.
5. The sample size seems adequate for this mixed methods study. The sample for the quantitative part of the study seemed adequate because a "significant drop in state anxiety was discovered after the visit, and satisfaction with the visit was exceedingly high" (Wendler et al., 2017, p. 45). This indicates that no Type II error occurred. In addition, extensive qualitative data were obtained to clearly address the purpose of the study.
6. The researchers did not address attrition
7. Nonprobability sampling method was used in the study.
8. Convenience sampling.
9. Generalization of findings is not the focus of this mixed methods feasibility study. Additionally, researchers noted "Generalizability of the study is hampered by the lack of a control group, and a convenience sample was used" (p. 56).
10. The setting was "a busy 19-bed PACU, where more than 1,200 hip and knee replacement surgeries were completed in 2011, in [a] level 1 trauma,

academically affiliated 500-bed Magnet hospital in the Midwest" (p. 48). This setting was a partially controlled environment as the researchers used curtains to maintain privacy and to facilitate the family visit in the PACU. Data were collected at the patient's bedside with the responsible staff nurse nearby.

CHAPTER 10—CLARIFYING MEASUREMENT AND DATA COLLECTION IN QUANTITATIVE RESEARCH

EXERCISE 1: TERMS AND DEFINITIONS

Measurement Concepts and Methods

1.	o	9.	d
2.	g	10.	c
3.	i	11.	a
4.	e	12.	n
5.	h	13.	f
6.	j	14.	b
7.	m	15.	l
8.	k		

Reliability, Validity, Accuracy, and Precision in Measurement

1.	n	8.	h
2.	a	9.	c
3.	l	10.	i
4.	e	11.	f
5.	m	12.	k
6.	g	13.	b
7.	d	14.	j

Data Collection

1.	c	4.	a
2.	d	5.	e
3.	b		

EXERCISE 2: LINKING IDEAS
1. ratio-level of measurement
2. 0.8
3. ordinal (The stages of breast cancer can be rank ordered according to level of severity.)
4. unequal; equal
5. a self-report form designed to elicit information through written, verbal, or electronic responses from study participants
6. Cronbach alpha
7. reliable; New scales with a Cronbach alpha of 0.70 are considered reliable (Grove & Cipher, 2017; Grove & Gray, 2019). As a scale is used in additional studies, the reliability will be examined and items will be revised as needed to improve the reliability and validity of the scale.
8. it is not valid

9. interval
10. reliability and validity
11. unstructured
12. structured
13. personal interview
14. predictive validity and concurrent validity
15. You might have listed any of the following or might have another idea that results in measurement error.
    a. Scale or questionnaire items lack reliability.
    b. Poorly developed scale or questionnaire that lacks validity.
    c. Scale lacks reliability or validity testing in the study population.
    d. Physiological measure that lacks precision in the measurement of a study variable.
    e. Physiological measure that lacks accuracy in the measurement of a study variable.
    f. Physiological equipment are not maintained or recalibrated as recommended by the manufacturer.
    g. Study participants are unable to read and understand the items on a scale because the reading level is too high for them.
    h. Variations in administration of the measurement method. For example, the person taking the measurements may not use the same procedure every time.
    i. Study participants leaving an item blank accidentally on a measurement scale.
    j. Participants completing a paper-and-pencil scale accidentally marking the wrong space on the answer sheet.
    k. Participants misreading or misunderstanding an item on a measurement method.
    l. Hitting the wrong key when entering data into the computer.
    m. Disorganization during data entry into a computer.

Measurement Error

1. b
2. a
3. a
4. b
5. b

Levels of Measurement

1. c	11. d
2. a	12. a
3. d	13. b
4. b or c (degree or years of education)	14. d
	15. a
5. a	16. d
6. b	17. b
7. d	18. a
8. d	19. a
9. c	20. d
10. a	

Scales

1. a
2. c
3. b

Sensitivity and Specificity

1. Completion of the table on sensitivity and specificity.

Diagnostic Test Results	Disease Present	Disease Absent or Not Present
Positive test	a (true positive)	b (false positive)
Negative test	c (false negative)	d (true negative)

2. Formula for sensitivity: $a/(a + c)$ = True positive rate
3. Formula for specificity: $d/(b + d)$ = True negative rate

Sensitivity and Specificity of Colonoscopy Screening Tests

4. 50
5. $(50 \div 300) \times 100\% = 0.166 \times 100\% = 16.667\% = 16.67\%$
6. 40
7. $(40 \div 790) \times 100\% = 0.0506 \times 100\% = 5.06\%$
8. Sensitivity $= 250/(250 + 40) \times 100\% = 250/290 \times 100\% = 0.862 \times 100 = 86.2\%$
9. The sensitivity value is strong at 86.2% in identifying a patient with the disease.
10. Specificity $= 750/(50 + 750) \times 100\% = 750/800 \times 100\% = 0.9375 \times 100\% = 93.75\%$
11. Positive LR $=$ sensitivity $\div$ (100% – specificity)
12. Positive LR $= 86.2\% \div (100\% - 93.75\%) = 86.2\% \div 6.25\% = 13.792\% = 13.79\%$
13. The LR of 13.79% is strong to rule in a disease because it is >10, which indicates that the patient has the disease when the test is positive.
14. Negative LR $=$ (100% – sensitivity) $\div$ specificity
15. Negative LR $= (100\% - 86.2\%) \div 93.75\% = 13.8\% \div 93.75\% = 0.147 = 0.15$
16. The LR of 0.15 is fairly strong to rule out a disease because it is close to the value of <0.1 that indicates the likelihood that the patient does not have the disease when the test is negative.

EXERCISE 3: WEB-BASED INFORMATION AND RESOURCES

1. http://www.qualitymeasures.ahrq.gov/
2. You might have identified one of the following websites or others that discuss the CES-R: http://cesd-r.com/; http://cesd-r.com/cesdr/

3. You might have identified one of the following websites or another one:
   https://www.brightfutures.org/mentalhealth/pdf/professionals/bridges/ces_dc.pdf
   http://www.ncbi.nlm.nih.gov/pubmed/2301363

4. http://www.wongbakerfaces.org/

5. http://www.apa.org/pi/about/publications/caregivers/practice-settings/assessment/tools/trait-state.aspx.
   https://www.mindgarden.com/145-state-trait-anxiety-inventory-for-adults

EXERCISE 4: CONDUCTING CRITICAL APPRAISALS TO BUILD AN EVIDENCE-BASED PRACTICE
Hallas, Koslap-Petraco, and Fletcher (2017) Study

1. Hallas et al. (2017) study measurement methods and directness of measurement.

Variables	Measurement Methods	Direct or Indirect Measurement Method
Maternal confidence	Toddler Care Questionnaire (TCQ)	Indirect measure
Social-emotional development of toddlers	Brigance Toddler Screen	Indirect measure

2. Identify the reliability and validity of the following measurement methods in the Hallas et al. (2017) study.

Variables	Measurement Methods' Reliability and Validity
Maternal confidence	"*Instrument #1* You might have identified some of the key ideas covered in the following quote: "The Toddler Care Questionnaire (TCQ) (Gross & Rocissano, 1988, 1989) is a measure of maternal confidence for all mothers of toddlers between the ages of 12 and 36 months (Table 2). Thirty-seven item responses are scored from A to E and equated to the numbers 1 to 5. The range in total scores is from 37 to 185. Higher scores reflect greater maternal confidence. The TCQ instrument reliability is reported to be between 0.91 and 0.96 and test–retest reliability is 0.87" (Hallas et al., 2017, p. 36).
Social-emotional development of toddlers	"*Instrument #2* You might have identified some of the key ideas covered in the following quote: "The Brigance Toddler Screen (Brigance & Glascoe, 2002) was used for toddlers between the ages of 12 to 33 months old (Table 3). The Brigance screens for social-emotional skills and consists of 10 items. One point is given for each item the toddler is able to perform with a total score of 10 points possible. Higher scores are indicative of higher social-emotional development. Test–retest reliability for the Brigance Toddler Screen is reported at 0.98 to 0.99. Specificity for the Brigance toddler screen was reported as ranging from 85% to 86% and sensitivity ranged from 76% to 77%" (Hallas et al., 2017, p. 36).

3. Critical appraisal of the TCQ: Hallas et al. (2017) included the items on this scale in their research report and the items appear to be measuring maternal confidence (evidence of content validity). The scale is appropriate for the age of the toddlers in this study and consistently implemented with each mother, strengthening the scale's reliability and validity. This is a multi-item scale that has detailed scoring instructions that also promotes the reliability and validity of the scale for data collection in this study. The TCQ has strong internal reliability (0.91–0.96) and test–retest reality (0.87) from previous research. However, the reliability of the scale in this study should have been included.

This scale was developed in 1988 so additional validity information should be available. In addition, the discussion of this scale would have been strengthened by providing construct validity information and reading level for the TCQ.

4. Critical appraisal of the Brigance Toddler Screen: This 10-item scale is included in the study for review with details of the scoring process, which add to the reliability and content validity of the scale. The scale is also age appropriate for the participants in this study. The Brigance Toddler Screen has very strong test–retest reliability (0.98–0.99) and adequate sensitivity and specificity for determining the social-emotional skills of toddlers. The RNs and RAs consistently collected data with this tool in Hallas et al. (2017). Discussion of this tool would have been strengthened by examining its reliability in this study and adding additional validity information from previous research.

5. You might have identified some of the key ideas in the following quote of the Hallas et al. (2017) data collection process: "**Procedures**: Prior to recruiting subjects, the PI and Co-I [co-investigator] met with the physicians, NPs, RNs, and office staff at each site and trained the RNs and RAs on study recruitment process, subject eligibility, study interventions, and process for obtaining informed consent. Fliers were then posted in each practice site that agreed to permit the researchers to recruit and invite all mothers, eligible by inclusion criteria, and their respective toddlers to participate in the study. Each mother who volunteered to participate in the study provided written informed consent prior to enrollment in the study. After enrollment, each mother–toddler dyad was given a folder that had been randomized into either the treatment or control group using a computer-generated random numbers list created by the study biostatistician. All RNs and RAs were blinded to folder contents, as all folders were identical and the DVDs were all labeled with a code only known to the PI. The folders with the pre-test results were given to the PI and all participants' identifying information was removed from the folder to assure anonymity. Each folder only contained the randomized number for the participant dyads. The names of the participants and their randomized numbers were maintained in a separate secured file cabinet in the office of the PI. Data were collected from June 30, 2009 to September 30, 2010…

Randomization: Allocation Concealment Mechanism
The allocation sequence was concealed from the RNs and RAs enrolling and assessing participants at each study site… All participants completed the same study instruments, thus no information about the group assignment was known to the RNs or RAs. Since all participants watched a DVD privately, the participants did not know if they were assigned to the treatment or control (Table 4)" (Hallas et al., 2017, pp. 35–36).

6. Critical appraisal of the Hallas et al. (2017) data collection process: The researchers provided quality information about the data collection process. The intervention was consistently implemented by DVDs to the treatment and control groups. Participants and data collectors were blinded to group assignment reducing the potential for bias during the study. The TCQ was completed by the mothers in a consistent manner, and the RNs and RAs consistently collected data with the Brigance Toddler Screen as was presented earlier in the answers to Questions 2–4. The data collected were kept confidential, stored in a precise way to prevent error, and given to the PI for data entry into a statistical program.

Wendler, Smith, Ellenburg, Gill, Anderson, and Spiegel-Thayer (2017) Study

1. Wendler et al. (2017) measurement methods and directness of measurement.

Variable(s)	Measurement Method(s)	Direct or Indirect Measurement Method
State anxiety	Spielberger State-Trait Anxiety Inventory (STAI)	Indirect measure
Satisfaction with visit	Single-item rating scale developed for this study	Indirect measure

2. Wendler et al. (2017) reliability and validity for measurement methods.

Variables	Scales' Reliability and Validity Information From the Wendler et al. (2017) Study
State anxiety	You might have identified some of the ideas from the following quote: The STAI is "a valid and reliable tool. It has been developed for all ages, translated into several languages, and is written at the fourth-grade reading level. It consists of 20 questions, and answers are provided on a Likert scale of 1 to 4, with a range of possible scores being 20 to 80. Scores of 20 to 39 are considered of low state anxiety, 40 to 59 of moderate state anxiety, and 60 to 80 of high state anxiety. The tool is widely reported to be valid and reliable" (Wendler et al., 2017, p. 50). "Cronbach's alpha, which evaluates the internal consistency of a tool, was 0.92, supporting the tool's reliability in this study" (Wendler et al., 2017, p. 52).
Satisfaction with visit	"Patient and family satisfaction is an important outcome and was measured using a simple and unidimensional question, which was asked on the day of the visit and again, via telephone, during the optional follow-up interview. The question was provided verbally: 'On a scale of 0-4, with zero meaning not at all satisfied and four meaning the most satisfied I can be, how satisfied were you with your family visit'?"(Wendler et al., 2017, p. 50).

3. Critical appraisal of STAI: Wendler et al. (2017) detailed the structure and scoring for the STAI Likert scale. The reading level of the scale was at the fourth grade level, which facilitated patients and family members being able to read and understand the scale items. The STAI was reported to be valid and reliable but no specific information from previous research was provided to support this statement. The Cronbach alpha was very strong for the STAI for the entire sample at 0.92; however, knowing the reliability of the scale for both the patients and the family members would have strengthened the reliability discussion. The measurement discussion would have been much stronger with coverage of reliability and of types of validity (such as content and construct validity) from previous research.

4. Critical appraisal of rating scale: The rating scale to measure satisfaction with visit had no reported reliability or validity from previous research since it was developed for this study. No pilot testing was done with the single-item scale to see if it measures what it is supposed to measure. Satisfaction with visit is a complex concept that cannot be clearly measured with a one-item scale. This scale provides very limited information and questionable findings about this study variable.

5. Wendler et al. (2017) study: Precision and accuracy of the measurement of vital signs.

Variables	Measurement Method and Reported Precision and Accuracy in This Study
Vital signs (VSs)—Mean blood pressure and heart rate	"VSs are monitored routinely during the PACU [postanesthesia care unit] phase 1 recovery period in this setting using the Dräger Infinity Delta vital signs monitor. This has a 'motion-tolerant…algorithm which uses a step-deflation method. The monitors are placed on a calibrated simulator by the biomedical engineer for annually ensuring validity and reliability of results as recommended by the manufacturer, as described by a company representative, K. Rosholt, in an e-mail communication (April 2012)" (Wendler et al., 2017, p. 50).

6. Critical appraisal of the measurement of VSs: The precise, accurate Dräger Infinity Delta VSs monitor was used in this study. The monitors were calibrated based on the manufacturer's recommendations. This monitor is much more precise and accurate than other methods of measuring, recording, and analyzing mean arterial pressure (MAP) and heart rate (HR).

7. You might have identified some of the key ideas for the data collection process for Wendler et al. (2017) study from the following quote: "Research assistants who performed the data collection were highly experienced PACU registered nurses (RNs), educated in protocol implementation, and who accompanied the family member during the visit. Thus, the care nurse maintained responsibility for the patient, whereas the PACU RN research assistant maintained responsibility for the family member, in case of any untoward responses during the visit" (Wendler et al., 2017, p. 48).

"State anxiety was measured at baseline, with the patient in the PACU and family member in the conference room immediately before the family visit, and again, immediately after the visit. Patients and family members served as their own controls… Patient and family satisfaction was also measured immediately after the visit but not while in each other's presence. The second measure of patient/family satisfaction was obtained during the follow-up interview; most of the patients and family members were interviewed together; therefore, these postdischarge measures of satisfaction were each heard at the same time as the interviewer… Because there were concerns that family visits could disrupt patients' VSs, MAP and HR were monitored and recorded before, during, and after the visit. For evaluation of MAP and HR, patients served as their own controls" (Wendler et al., 2017, p. 50).

8. Wendler et al. (2017) provided a flow diagram in Figure 1 of the study participants' activities throughout the study. This diagram provided detail and clarity to the data collection process. The researchers also described the RAs as highly trained, experienced RNs, but they did not describe the training process or the interrater reliability achieved. The RNs provided structure for the visit to ensure consistency. The collection of data with the STAI, rating scale for satisfaction, and VSs monitor were clearly described and seemed appropriate for the study. The organized, structured data collection process promotes the collection of quality data that decreases the potential for error.

CHAPTER 11—UNDERSTANDING STATISTICS IN RESEARCH

EXERCISE 1: TERMS AND DEFINITIONS

1.	e	9.	b
2.	c	10.	f
3.	o	11.	g
4.	d	12.	k
5.	a	13.	l
6.	m	14.	h
7.	i	15.	j
8.	n		

EXERCISE 2: LINKING IDEAS

1. reduce and organize numerical data from a study to give it meaning
2. You might have listed any three of the following:
   a. manage missing data
   b. describe the sample and study variables
   c. examine reliability of measurement methods
   d. conduct exploratory data analysis to identify outliers
   e. conduct inferential statistical analysis
   f. conduct posthoc analyses if required
3. You might have listed any three of the following analysis techniques:
   a. Estimates of central tendency, such as mode, median, and mean
   b. Estimates of dispersion, such as range, variance, and standard deviation
   c. Examination of data to identify outliers
   d. Frequencies and percentages are calculated for nominal and ordinal data to determine the occurrence of demographic variables. For example, with a sample size of 250, the sample was 128 (51.2%) female and 122 (48.8%) male.
   e. Differences among groups are examined to demonstrate equivalence at the start of the study.
4. a. significant and predicted results
   b. nonsignificant results
   c. significant and unpredicted results
   d. mixed results
   e. unexpected results
5. You might have listed any of the following:
   a. findings
   b. significance of findings
   c. clinical importance of findings
   d. comparison of the findings from the current study to the findings from previous studies
   e. limitations
   f. conclusions
   g. generalization of findings
   h. implications for nursing
   i. recommendations for further study

6. The normal curve is a symmetrical curve where the mean, median, and mode fall at the same point. Figure 11-1 in Chapter 11 of your textbook, *Understanding Nursing Research*, 7th edition, includes a drawing of the normal curve with a mean of 0 and a standard deviation of 1.
7. 95%
8. one-tailed test of significance
9. Type I error
10. group differences
11. mode
12. standard deviation
13. the group size
14. scatterplot
15. bivariate analysis

Linking Statistics With Analysis Techniques

1. j
2. f
3. g
4. a
5. d
6. c
7. h
8. e
9. b
10. i

Linking Levels of Measurement With Analysis Techniques

1. c
2. a
3. c
4. c
5. a and b
6. b
7. c
8. c
9. c
10. b and c
11. a
12. a and b
13. c
14. c
15. a and b

Statements, Inferences, and Generalizations

1. d
2. b
3. a
4. c

Describing the Sample

1. Age in years
2. Associate's Degree in Nursing (ADN)
3. 40–49 years
4. Standard deviation $(SD) = 2.1$
5. 35 years of experience that is identified in the range
6. $95\% = \text{Mean} \pm 1.96(SD) = 15.5 \pm 1.96(2.1) = 15.5 \pm 4.12 = (11.38, 19.62)$

Measures of Central Tendency

1. 3.42
2. 3.10

3. 3.00 because this score is the most frequent value (mode) in this distribution of scores.
4. $\text{Mean} \pm SD = 3.42 + 0.76 = 4.18$ and $3.42 - 0.76 = 2.66$
   2.66 to 4.18 or (2.66, 4.18)

Name That Statistical Analysis Technique!

1. d—Analysis of variance (ANOVA) is conducted to determine group differences for three or more groups; interval or ratio level data
2. a—Chi-square analysis is conducted to determine whether two variables are independent or related in a study; nominal level data
3. c—Pearson correlation is conducted to examine relationships between variables in a study; interval or ratio level data
4. b—*t*-test is conducted to determine a difference between two groups in a study; interval or ratio level data

Significance of Results

1. NS
2. *
3. *
4. NS
5. *

EXERCISE 3: WEB-BASED INFORMATION AND RESOURCES

1. The following websites address power analysis calculation and you might have identified other sites for power analysis:
   a. http://power-analysis.com/ *Power and Precision* provides free software to calculate power analysis.
   b. http://powerandsamplesize.com/ *Free, Online, Easy-to-Use Power and Sample Size Calculators*
   c. *DSS Research Calculators*: https://www.dssresearch.com/KnowledgeCenter/toolkitcalculators/statisticalpowercalculators.aspx
   d. *Making sense of statistical power*: https://www.americannursetoday.com/making-sense-of-statistical-power/
2. SPSS stands for Statistical Package for the Social Sciences
3. You might have identified one of the following websites or another that addresses introduction to SPSS:
   a. Social Science Computing Cooperative (SSCC): http://ssc.wisc.edu/sscc/pubs/spss/classintro/spss_students1.html
   b. How to use SPSS to analyze data at https://www.wikihow.com/Analyse-Data-Using-SPSS

c.   Introduction to SPSS on YouTube: https://www.youtube.com/watch?v=msI7xf0tInE

4.   You can locate the Grove and Cipher (2017) *Statistics for Nursing Research* (2nd ed.) text published by Elsevier at the following website: https://www.elsevier.com/books/statistics-for-nursing-research/grove/978-0-323-35881-1

Amazon also provides a website for the text: https://www.amazon.com/Statistics-Nursing-Research-Workbook-Evidence-Based/dp/0323358810

5.   a.   Descriptive statistics conducted to describe the sample included frequencies, percentages, mean, standard deviation, and range. Review the Study Results section in the article (Coleman, 2017, pp. 139–140).

b.   Inferential statistical analyses included Pearson correlation (Table 1) and stepwise multiple regression.

c.   Bivariate Pearson correlation is conducted to examine relationships between two variables and the results of these correlations are presented in Table 1. Regression analysis involves using the independent or predictor variables to predict the dependent variable of depressive symptoms in this study.

d.   Coleman (2017, p. 141) recommended investigating "how changes in HRQOL [health related quality of life] affect African American men and women living with HIV/AIDS from a longitudinal perspective. Longitudinal data would provide a more comprehensive understanding about the clinical trajectory that changes in HRQOL have on depressive symptoms overtime."

EXERCISE 4: CONDUCTING CRITICAL APPRAISALS TO BUILD AN EVIDENCE-BASED PRACTICE

Hallas, Koslap-Petraco, and Fletcher (2017) Study

1.   The study included two groups: a treatment group and a control group.

2.   Study participants were randomly assigned to the treatment and control groups.

3.   Independent groups because the participants were randomly assigned to the groups.

4.   Link of variables, level of measurement, and descriptive data analysis techniques:

Demographic and Study Variables	Level of Measurement	Descriptive Analysis Techniques
Race/Ethnicity	Nominal	Frequency, percentage
Occasional help from babysitter	Nominal	Frequency, percentage
Toddler goes to day care	Nominal	Frequency, percentage
Other children in the home	Nominal	Frequency, percentage
Mother works full or part time	Nominal	Frequency, percentage
Mother's age (years)	Ratio	Mean, standard deviation
Baby's age (months)	Ratio	Mean, standard deviation
Toddler Care Questionnaire (TCQ) scores at baseline (pretest) and post-test results	Interval*	Mean, standard deviation
Brigance Toddler Screen scores at baseline (pretest) and post-test results	Interval*	Mean, standard deviation

*Multi-item scales such as the TCQ and Brigance Toddler Screen are considered to have interval level data (see Chapter 10; Grove & Gray, 2019).

5.   a.   Only the mother's age (years) characteristic was significantly different between the treatment and control groups at the beginning of the study. All other characteristics and pretest baseline scores for the TCQ and Brigance were not significantly different (Table 6; Hallas et al., 2017, p. 38).

    b. This is a study strength that indicates the groups were similar for most variables at the beginning of the study.

    c. Thus, any significant changes at the completion of the study are more likely to be caused by the study treatment or intervention rather than original group differences (Grove & Cipher, 2017). However, the mothers in the treatment group were significantly younger than those in the control group, which might have affected the study results.

6. Inferential statistics conducted for the analysis of the TCQ and Brigance scores were mixed regression models to examine change over time in outcomes measures (TCQ and Brigance) (Hallas et al., 2017, p. 38). Mixed models were conducted to examine differences between pretest and post-test for both the treatment group and the control group (Tables 7 and 8; Hallas et al., 2017, p. 39). Differences were also examined between the TCQ and Brigance post-test scores for the treatment and control groups.

7. The treatment group had a significant improvement ($p = 0.002$) from pretest to post-test for the TCQ; the control group did not show significant improvement ($p = 0.103$) (see Table 7). The DVD parenting skills intervention did show a significant improvement in the treatment group but there was no significant difference between the post-tests for the control and treatment groups. The researchers reported that the study limitations might have affected these results and additional research is needed to test the effectiveness of the intervention.

8. "Hypothesis one was not supported. Toddlers in both the treatment and control groups improved in their performance on the Brigance toddler screen over the 3-month study period… The second hypothesis was supported. The results showed a significant difference for the treatment group of mother–toddler dyads in the mothers' maternal confidence in caring for toddlers as measured by the TCQ" (Hallas et al., 2017, p. 39). The control group received a DVD of nutritional information and the treatment group a DVD of parenting skills. Both groups receiving information might have caused the improvement in the treatment and control groups, resulting in nonsignificant findings.

9. a. Yes, the *t*-test value of 2.079 is statistically significant since $p = 0.042$ is smaller than the level of significance (alpha) that was set at 0.05 for the study.

    b. Yes, this result is clinically important since it shows the "Mothers in the treatment group were significantly younger than the mothers in the control group" (Hallas et al., 2017, p. 38), which

could have contributed to the nonsignificant findings between the treatment and control groups. This study requires replication with a larger sample before findings are generalized.

10. "The generalizability of this study is limited due to the small sample size that limited the statistical power of this study. Replication of this study using a larger study sample may be beneficial as there are few rigorously conducted RCTs investigating the social-emotional development of toddlers.

    While we followed a rigorous approach for randomization of study participants, mothers in the treatment group were significantly younger than those in the control group which may have affected the level of confidence of the mothers prior to the treatment based on maternal age. Even though we used five different primary care settings within culturally diverse populations, we had a greater representation of white and Latino families in some of the practice settings, therefore, African American families may have been underrepresented" (Hallas et al., 2017, pp. 39–40).

    Yes, the significantly younger mothers in the intervention group, small sample size, limited statistical power of the study, and the limited diversity of the sample helped explain the nonsignificant findings.

11. The researchers indicated that the DVD might be used in pediatric primary care settings because of the potential benefit and limited risks. However, they recommended additional research to determine the effectiveness of the parenting skills DVD. "Pediatric nurses and nurse practitioners are encouraged to replicate this study in primary care offices to provide the same level of care for mother-toddler dyads and to share their outcomes on changes in maternal confidence and toddler social-emotional development. Doctor of Nursing Practice (DNP) graduates and/or students may want to consider implementing a quality improvement study using this educational intervention to determine the effect on maternal confidence and toddler social-emotional development" (Hallas et al., 2017, p. 39).

    Thus, either answers of using the intervention in practice now or recommending additional research before use in practice are acceptable.

Wendler, Smith, Ellenburg, Gill, Anderson, and Spiegel-Thayer (2017) Study

1. Link of variables, level of measurement, and descriptive analysis techniques (Table 1, Wendler et al. (2017, p. 52).

Demographic Variables	Level of Measurement	Descriptive Analysis Techniques
Patient and family member's age (years)	Ratio	Mean (*M*), standard deviation (*SD*), range
Patient and family member's race	Nominal	Frequency, percentage
Patient and family member's gender	Nominal	Frequency, percentage

2. This was a "descriptive, single-group, and mixed-methods study" (Wendler et al., 2017, p. 47).
3. The scores were paired or dependent since they were pretest and post-test scores for a single group. The researchers examined differences in state anxiety scores before and after the family member visit for both patients and family members, so they served as their own control in the pretest.
4. "Repeated-samples (paired or dependent samples) *t*-tests were used to calculated the state anxiety responses of patients and their family members. Table 2 illustrates the patients and family members' mean STAI before and after the visit indicating a clinically and statically significant reduction in state anxiety after the visit (p < .001)" (Wendler et al., 2017, p. 52). Yes, the repeated or dependent *t*-tests are appropriate since the patients' and family members' pretests are serving as the control for each group. There is not an official control group in this study as a basis of comparison, making this a descriptive study design as indicated in the answer to Question 2.
5. a. Yes, the *t*-test value of 5.63 is statistically significant since *p* < .001 is smaller than the level of significance (alpha) that is usually set at 0.05 for most nursing studies.
    b. This result demonstrates a significant decrease in the state anxiety responses of the patients after the family member visit. This is a clinically important outcome for the patient that might improve satisfaction for the patients and family members and facilitate recovery for the patients.
6. a. The MBP and HR were analyzed with mean *(M)* and standard deviation *(SD),* and repeated-measures analysis of variance (ANOVA).
    b. Yes, these descriptive and inferential statistics were appropriate since the MBP and HR are

ratio-level data described by *M* and *SD*. The MBP and HR were collected at three intervals so an ANOVA was conducted to detect differences in the repeated measures of MBPs and HRs in this study.

7. a. No, the MBPs and HRs were not significantly different at baseline, beginning of the visit, and end of the visit for the patients as indicated in Table 3 (Wendler, 2017, p. 53).
    b. The MBP result was $F = 0.56$, $p = .573$ and HR result was $F = 0.356$, $p = .702$. Since the *p* values are greater than $\alpha = 0.05$, the results are nonsignificant.
8. The researchers limited the generalization of the study findings as indicated by the following quote: "Generalizability of the study is hampered by the lack of a control group, and a convenience sample was used. We did not obtain any information about those potential patients who declined inclusion into the study, so it is unknown whether there were differences between those who self-selected into the study and those who did not" (Wendler et al., 2017, p. 56).
9. You could have identified key conclusions from the following quote: "Family visitation in the PACU is safe and effectively reduces anxiety; it also may improve the perception of waiting and may drive patient and family satisfaction on the day of the surgery. Although not every patient or family member may choose to visit during the early recovery period, this study, and others, provide the scientific basis for promoting family visits during phase 1 recovery. This study demonstrated the feasibility of phase 1 visits, and results provide further support for instituting family visits to reduce anxiety and enhance patient satisfaction when patients and family members agree" (Wendler et al., 2017, p. 56).
    Yes, the conclusions seem appropriate based on the significant findings for the state anxiety levels for both patients and family members. However, additional research is needed with stronger design, such as a RCT with a control group, protocol for the intervention, and a larger sample size to determine the effectiveness of the intervention.
10. Both patient and designated family member responded "to the semistructured interview questions at the same time" (Wendler et al., 2017, p. 49),
11. **"Phase *II*: Qualitative Results**
    The final data reduction resulted in the identification of 14 categories, which described the content, and the overarching theme emerged. Only seven secondary codes did not fit within the final structure... Categories with examples from the data that support the categories appear in Table 4" (Wendler et al., 2017, p. 52).

CHAPTER 12—CRITICAL APPRAISAL OF QUANTITATIVE AND QUALITATIVE RESEARCH FOR NURSING PRACTICE

EXERCISE 1: TERMS AND DEFINITIONS
1. e
2. d
3. f
4. c
5. b
6. a

EXERCISE 2: LINKING IDEAS
1. strengths, weaknesses (limitations), meaning, and significance
2. You might include any three of the following:
   a. What are the major strengths of the study?
   b. What are the major weaknesses or limitations of the study?
   c. Are the findings of the study an accurate reflection of reality?
   d. What is the significance of the findings for nursing?
   e. Are the findings consistent with those of previous studies?
3. You might list any of the following or have other ideas:
   a. Critically appraise studies for class assignments.
   b. Critically appraise research to share the findings with other healthcare professionals.
   c. Read and critically appraise studies to solve a problem in practice.
   d. Critically appraise studies in a selected area and summarize the findings for use in practice.
   e. Critically appraise a proposed study to determine whether it is ethical to conduct in your clinical agency.
4. rights, informed consent
5. a. Purpose
   b. Qualitative approach
   c. Sample
   d. Key results

Determination of Quantitative Study Strengths and Weaknesses
1. W
2. S
3. W
4. W
5. S
6. S
7. W or S. Weakness (W) if the goal of sampling was to recruit a heterogeneous sample representing the target population. Network sampling could be a strength (S) if the sample was difficult to recruit because the topic was sexual abuse or other sensitive or stigmatized topics. In such cases, network sampling might be the only feasible strategy for recruiting an adequate number of participants.
8. S
9. W
10. S
11. W
12. S
13. S
14. W
15. S

Determination of Qualitative Study Strengths and Weaknesses
1. S
2. W
3. W
4. S
5. S
6. W
7. S
8. W
9. S
10. S
11. S
12. W
13. S
14. W
15. S

EXERCISE 3: WEB-BASED INFORMATION AND RESOURCES
1. The QSEN website for pre-licensure nursing students is: http://qsen.org/competencies/pre-licensure-ksas/
2. The six QSEN competency areas are:
   a. Patient-centered care
   b. Teamwork and collaboration
   c. Evidence-based practice (EBP)
   d. Quality improvement (QI)
   e. Safety
   f. Informatics
3. Evidence-based practice (EBP)
4. EBP Attitude: "Appreciate strengths and weaknesses of scientific bases [studies] for practice" QSEN (2017). QSEN competencies: Retrieved from http://qsen.org/competencies/pre-licensure-ksas/
5. EBP Skill: "Read original research and evidence reports related to area of practice" QSEN (2017). QSEN competencies: Retrieved from http://qsen.org/competencies/pre-licensure-ksas/
6. The Magnet Recognition Program website is: https://www.nursingworld.org/organizational-programs/magnet/
7. Website to find agencies with Magnet status is: https://www.nursingworld.org/organizational-programs/magnet/find-a-magnet-facility/

EXERCISE 4: CONDUCTING CRITICAL APPRAISALS TO BUILD AN EVIDENCE-BASED PRACTICE

Conduct the critical appraisals of the two studies—Hallas, Koslap-Petraco, and Fletcher (2017) and Erikson and Davies (2017)—which are included in Appendices A and B of this study guide. Review the answers to the critical appraisal exercises for Chapters 1 through 11 to assist yourself in these critical appraisals. Ask your instructor to clarify any questions that you might have. Additionally, an example critique summary, which corresponds to question 1. v. for the Hallas et al. (2017) study, is provided below.

Overall, the Hallas et al. (2017) article was detailed, well organized, and clearly written. Researchers created a highly controlled study by using a consistent DVD intervention that reduced possibility of intervention variation, group randomization and concealment of group allocation to participants and researchers (double blind), and five comparable pediatric primary healthcare settings. The Toddler Care Questionnaire (TCQ) and the Brigance Toddler Screen used for measurement of the study variables have strong documented reliability from previous studies. However, the reliability values of these scales were not included for this study. In addition, the researchers did not discuss the validity of these two scales from previous research. However, they did provide the items for the scales so the content validity of the scales might be examined.

The fairly high sample attrition caused the study to have low statistical power (less than 30 in both the treatment and control groups), which might have contributed to selected nonsignificant findings. Both the control and the treatment groups improved so there might have been a maturation affect that biased the study results. Both groups received a DVD educational program that might have affected their scores on the study instruments.

The study appears to be ethical. Hallas et al. (2017) indicated that IRB approval and informed consent for the mother–toddler dyads were obtained. The risks were minimal and the potential benefits were strong, which resulted in a positive benefit-risk ratio.

The three authors demonstrate strong educational, research, and clinical expertise for conducting this study. The researchers indicated that the DVD might be used in pediatric primary care settings because of the potential benefit and limited risk. However, they recommended additional research to determine the effectiveness of the parenting skills DVD. The researchers' recommendations are appropriate based on the study findings.

CHAPTER 13—BUILDING AN EVIDENCE-BASED NURSING PRACTICE

EXERCISE 1: TERMS AND DEFINITIONS

1.	h	8.	j
2.	a	9.	d
3.	m	10.	i
4.	b	11.	g
5.	e	12.	n
6.	k	13.	c
7.	l	14.	f

EXERCISE 2: LINKING IDEAS

1. Evidence-based nursing practice promotes desired outcomes for patients, nurses, and healthcare agencies. You might have identified any of the following benefits (or others) for nurses to implement evidence-based practice (EBP):
   a. Improves quality of care delivered by nurses in a variety of healthcare settings.
   b. Improves patient outcomes such as decreased signs and symptoms, improved functional status, improved physical and psychological health, prevention of illnesses, and promotion of health through implementation of healthy lifestyles.
   c. Promotes the delivery of safe care.
   d. Promotes the delivery of cost-effective care.
   e. Decreases need for healthcare services.
   f. Decreases patient recovery time.
   g. Improves the work environment for nurses, increases their productivity, and promotes quality outcomes for patients and nurses.
   h. Accomplishes a Quality and Safety Education for Nurses (QSEN) competency focused on promoting EBP for nursing programs and students.
   i. Increases patient and family satisfaction with care.
   j. Important to meet accreditation requirements.
   k. Important for a healthcare agency to achieve Magnet status.
   l. Increases access to care by providing different types of healthcare agencies and services with a variety of healthcare providers.
2. You might have identified any of the following:
   a. Read research journals in nursing and other healthcare disciplines.
   b. Read clinical journals with a major focus on publishing research articles.

   c. Use evidence-based websites, such as the Agency for Healthcare Research and Quality (AHRQ) and many others that communicate evidence-based guidelines and reference a variety of research publications. (Table 13.1, Evidence-Based Practice Resources, in Chapter 13 of your textbook, *Understanding Nursing Research*, 7th edition, identifies several resources.)

   d. Attend professional nursing meetings and conferences to obtain information on current studies, research syntheses, and evidence-based guidelines for practice.

   e. Attend nursing research conferences for current study findings and to promote collaboration in research activities.

   f. Participate in collaborative groups of nurses and other healthcare professionals that share research findings in your clinical agencies.

   g. Note study findings reported on television and on the Internet.

   h. Read research findings reported in newspapers and popular journals.

3. You might have identified any of the following challenges to EBP in nursing:

   a. Nursing lacks the research evidence in certain areas for the implementation of EBP.

   b. There is a concern that research evidence generated based on population data might not transfer to the care of individual patients who respond in unique ways.

   c. The best research evidence is currently generated mainly from quantitative and outcomes research methodologies, and more work is needed to synthesize qualitative research and determine its contribution to EBP.

   d. The EBP movement might lead to the development of evidence-based guidelines that provide a narrow, specific approach that limits the care provided by healthcare providers.

   e. Healthcare agencies and administrators do not provide the resources to support the implementation of EBP by nurses.

4. You might have identified any of the following:

   a. EBP requires the synthesis of research evidence from randomized controlled trials, and these types of studies are limited in nursing.

   b. Researchers have found limited association between nursing interventions/processes and patient outcomes in acute care settings.

   c. There is significant variation in the methods to measure the effect of independent variables (nursing interventions) on patient outcomes.

   d. There is a need for additional studies to determine the effectiveness of nursing interventions.

   e. More replication studies are needed to strengthen the knowledge in significant areas of nursing practice.

   f. There is a need to identify areas where research evidence is needed for practice.

   g. Nurses need to be more active in conducting quality syntheses (systematic reviews, meta-analyses, meta-syntheses, and mixed methods systematic reviews) of research evidence in selected areas.

5. You might have identified any two of the following triggers for EBP in clinical agencies or others that you might know:

   a. Clinical or patient identified issue

   b. Organization, state, or national initiative

   c. Data/new evidence

   d. Accrediting agency requirements/regulations

   e. Philosophy of care

6. a. Immediate use—using research-based intervention in practice exactly as it was developed.

   b. Reinvention—occurs when the research intervention is modified to meet the needs of a healthcare agency or nurses within the agency.

   c. Cognitive change—occurs when nurses incorporate research findings into their knowledge bases and use this information to defend a point, write agency protocols or policies, or develop a clinical paper for presentation or publication.

7. Table 13.1 in Chapter 13 of your textbook, *Understanding Nursing Research*, 7th edition, provides several EBP resources.

   a. National Guideline Clearinghouse website (www.guideline.gov), which includes integrative reviews of research. This website was initiated by the Agency for Healthcare Research and Quality (AHRQ).

   b. Cochrane Library, which includes systematic reviews, meta-analyses, and integrative reviews of research to determine the best research evidence in selected practice areas. The Cochrane Reviews are available at http://www.cochrane.org and then search for research reviews.

   c. Cochrane Nursing Care Field (CNCF) is included as part of the Cochrane Collaboration and supports the conduct, dissemination, and use of systemic reviews in nursing. The CNCF is available at http://cncf.cochrane.org/.

   d. The National Library of Health is located in the United Kingdom (UK); you can search for evidence-based sources using the following website: http://www.evidence.nhs.uk/.

   e. The National Institute for Health and Clinical Excellence (NICE) was organized in the United Kingdom to provide access to current EBP guidelines; it can be accessed at http://nice.org.uk/.

f. The Joanna Briggs Institute is an international evidence-based organization in Australia that provides access to numerous evidence-based summaries. You can search the Joanna Briggs Institute website at http://joannabriggs.org/.

g. The Nursing Reference Center (NRC) includes a collection of evidence-based care sheets that provide best practice for interventions and clinical conditions. The NRC requires a subscription, so check with your librarian.

h. Meta-analyses and systematic reviews: Search CINAHL and MEDLINE for these types of research syntheses.

i. Meta-syntheses and mixed methods systematic reviews: Search CINAHL and MEDLINE for these types of research syntheses. You might also search for integrative reviews of research using these search engines.

8. Formal and informal evaluations of outcomes for the following groups:
    a. patients, families, and communities
    b. nurses and other healthcare professionals
    c. administrators and healthcare agencies

9. feasibility, current practice

10. a. Use research evidence in practice.
    b. Consider using research knowledge in practice.
    c. Do not use the research findings in practice.

11. use of research evidence in practice or the use of evidence-based guidelines in practice.

12. Evidence-Based Practice Centers (EPCs)

Understanding Research Syntheses

1.	d	9.	a,b,c,d
2.	a,b,c,d	10.	c
3.	c	11.	d
4.	a	12.	b
5.	a, b	13.	c
6.	c	14.	a,b,c,d
7.	a	15.	a,b
8.	b		

Application of the Phases of Stetler's Model

1.	c	4.	b
2.	d	5.	e
3.	a		

Application of the Iowa Model of Evidence-Based Practice

1.	e	4.	f
2.	c	5.	d
3.	a	6.	b

Agency's Readiness for Evidence-Based Practice

Obtain the answers to these questions by gathering information in the agency where you are doing your clinical hours this semester. Ask your faculty if these questions might be covered in class or on the discussion board.

1. Review some of the protocols, algorithms, policies, and guidelines in the unit where you are doing clinical and note if the policies are documented with research sources. If these documents are without references, you cannot assume they are based on current research.

2. The policies, protocols, algorithms, and guidelines might be based on the knowledge and experience of the nurses developing them and research articles, but not documented with research references or evidence-based websites.

3. Are there nurses in the agency who are responsible for developing and revising policies, protocols, algorithms, and guidelines, and educating nurses to make the necessary changes in practice? Is there a team of nurses working toward meeting accreditation and Magnet status guidelines? These individuals are often the change agents in an agency and promote the use of evidence-based protocols, algorithms, policies, and guidelines in practice.

4. Ask the staff about access to a library in the agency. Do they have Internet access or hard copies of journals, and what are the names of the journals? Are these research journals or clinical journals with research articles? Do the nurses have access to evidence-based websites on the computers in the agency?

5. Read the mission and goals of the clinical agency. Ask nurses about the goal of EBP in their agency. What steps have been taken to promote EBP?

6. The healthcare agencies that currently have Magnet status can be viewed online at the American Nurses Credentialing Center (ANCC) website at https://wwwnursingworld.org/organizational-programs/magnet/. Look on this website for the status of the agency. If the agency has Magnet status, how do they document the outcomes of care in their agency to maintain this status? If the agency is seeking Magnet status, where are they in the process of obtaining this designation? Having Magnet status indicates the agency has a commitment to EBP and excellence in nursing care.

7. "The aim [purpose] of this study was to assess a demonstration project intended to pilot and evaluate a structured EBP education with mentoring innovation for nurses in a multi-hospital system" (Friesen, Brady, Milligan, & Christensen, 2017, p. 22).

You might share this source with nurses in the clinical agencies where you are completing clinical hours.

EXERCISE 3: WEB-BASED INFORMATION AND RESOURCES

1. AHRQ National Guideline Clearinghouse website to search for evidence-based guideline summaries by clinical specialty is: https://www.guideline.gov/browse/clinical-specialty
2. ONS EBP guidelines for managing anxiety: https://www.ons.org/practice-resources/pep/anxiety
   The EBP information on anxiety was current since it was updated April 3, 2017.
3. CNCF Cochran Resources in Nursing website is: http://nursingcare.cochrane.org/resources
4. NRC Patient Education Reference Center website is: https://www.ebscohost.com/nursing/products/patient-education-reference-center
5. U.S. Preventive Services Task Force Recommendations: Information for consumers' website is: https://www.uspreventiveservicestaskforce.org/Tools/ConsumerInfo/Index/information-for-consumers
6. The website for *Healthy People 2020* is https://www.healthypeople.gov/
7. The website for Genomics can be found at: https://www.healthypeople.gov/2020/topics-objectives/topic/genomics

EXERCISE 4: CONDUCTING CRITICAL APPRAISALS TO BUILD AN EVIDENCE-BASED PRACTICE

1. "The objective of the present study was to conduct a systematic review and meta-analysis to evaluate the effects of massage therapy on acute postoperative pain among adult thoracic surgery patients in the ICU and early post-ICU discharge compared to usual care or compared to sham massage or attention control" (Boitor et al., 2017, p. 340). This objective was clearly and concisely presented and directed the methodology of the research synthesis.
2. "The meta-analysis was reported per the Preferred Reporting Items for Systematic Reviews and Meta-Analysis statement [PRISMA] (Liberati et al., 2009)" (Boitor et al., 2017, p. 304). This strengthens the research synthesis since the PRISMA format is the internationally recommended format for reporting meta-analyses.
3. The PICOS format was not identified in this research synthesis but would have included the following content:
   - Population: Critically and acutely ill adult thoracic surgery patients
   - Intervention: Massage or massage with analgesia
   - Comparison of groups: Massage (intervention) group versus active control, massage versus standard care; massage versus active control, versus standard care (Figure 1, Boitor et al., 2017, p. 342).
   - Outcome: Acute postoperative pain
   - Study design: RCTs
4. A detailed description of the rigorous literature search was provided on page 340 of the article under the heading *Search Strategy*. "Eligible studies were identified by searching MEDLINE, Embase, CINAHL, PsycInfo, Web of Science, Scopus, and the Cochrane Central Register of Controlled Trials… The search strategy was developed with assistance of a research librarian who conducted the search… Authors of the included trials were contacted to attempt to identify any unpublished trials" (Boitor et al., 2017, p. 340).
5. a. "The database and registry searches and manual searches of reference lists retrieved 194 total citations, including 165 unique citations…".
   b. 25 underwent full-text reviews.
   c. "12 were determined to be eligible and were included" (Boitor et al., 2017, p. 340).
   d. The details of this selection process are presented in Figure 1. Literature Search and Study Selection flow diagram recommended in the PRISMA format (Boitor et al., 2017, p. 342).
6. The characteristics of the 12 studies were examined and presented in Table 1 (Boitor et al., 2017, p. 343). The qualities of the 12 studies were detailed and the risk of bias within the studies was addressed (Boitor et al, 2017, pp. 341–342). The authors might have provided more details on their critical appraisal of the studies and the format that they used for this process.
7. Yes, a meta-analysis was conducted on the results from the seven studies and these results are presented in Figure 3 (Boitor et al., 2017, p. 344).
8. Boitor et al., 2017, p. 339) concluded: "Massage, in addition to pharmacological analgesia, reduces acute post-cardiac surgery pain intensity."
9. No, massage was not considered clinically significant in reducing cardiac surgery patients' pain as indicated by the following quote: "Massage can complement pharmacological analgesia in reducing postoperative pain by almost 1 point on a 0-10 scale in both critically and acutely ill cardiac surgery patients. Although this does not reach the clinically significant 2-point reduction in acute pain intensity, it appears to be safe and may have the potential to

concomitantly improve other symptoms such as pain distress and anxiety" (Boitor et al., 2017, p. 344.).

Additional Evidence-Based Practice Projects

1. Use the content in Chapter 13 of your textbook, *Understanding Nursing Research*, 7th edition, to implement an EBP project guided by Stetler's Model (textbook Figure 13.2) or the Iowa Evidence-Based Model (textbook Figure 13.3).
2. Use the Grove Model in textbook Figure 13.4 to direct the implementation of the evidence-based guidelines.

CHAPTER 14—INTRODUCTION TO ADDITIONAL RESEARCH METHODOLOGIES IN NURSING: MIXED METHODS AND OUTCOMES RESEARCH

EXERCISE 1: TERMS AND DEFINITIONS

1. j
2. l
3. m
4. k
5. a
6. h
7. g
8. n
9. f
10. i
11. q
12. c
13. p
14. d
15. o
16. b
17. e

EXERCISE 2: LINKING IDEAS

Key Ideas for Mixed Methods Research

1. Convergent concurrent, exploratory sequential, explanatory sequential
2. pragmatic
3. The answers could be any of the following: (1) Mixed methods studies often require a team of researchers with different backgrounds and abilities. Developing a proposal with a team may require more time to come to agreement on a research plan; (2) For some designs, one phase of the study must be completed and the data analyzed before the second phase is implemented, which requires additional time; (3) Mixed methods studies often involve more data to be analyzed, requiring more time; (4) Two types of data must be analyzed and then integrated for an additional level of meaning.
4. qualitative
5. Parallel design
6. Correct answers are any of the following: (1) The research topic is significant; (2) The research team combined has the expertise to complete all the

methods of the study and integrate the findings; (3) The mixed methods study design and methods are appropriate for the purpose of the study; (4) The participants in the study can provide the rich data needed to answer the research question; (5) The methods of the study were implemented according to standards of rigor; (6) The findings of two study components were integrated in a meaningful way using description, figures, or tables; (7) The conclusions and implications were appropriately cautious in the light of the study's limitations; (8) The study contributed to the knowledge base of nursing.

Key Ideas for Outcomes Research

1. Donabedian
2. a. Physical–psychological function
   b. Psychological function
   c. Social function
3. a. Structure: Nursing units, hospitals, clinics, or home health agencies
   b. Process: What care is provided or practice patterns of interventions provided patients. How care is provided or practice style and standards of care delivered (clinical guidelines, critical paths, or care maps)
   c. Outcomes: Morbidity rates, mortality rates, length of stay in hospitals, complications from procedures, side effects of medications, medication errors, fall rates, infection rates, costs, or patient satisfaction
4. nursing-sensitive outcomes
5. assessment, nursing diagnosis, nurse-initiated interventions
6. communication, case management, coordination of care, continuity, monitoring
7. outcome
8. a. Clinical guidelines
   b. Critical paths
   c. Care maps
9. heterogeneous
10. You might have listed any of the following questions:
    a. What are the end results of patients' care (all care provided by all care providers)?
    b. What effect does nursing care (all care by all nurses) have on the end results of patients' care?
    c. Are there some nursing acts that have no effect at all on outcomes or that actually cause harm?
    d. Can we measure and thus identify the end results of nursing care?
    e. How do we distinguish care provided by nurses from care provided by other professionals in examining patient outcomes?

    f. When do we measure the effects of care (end results) (e.g., change in symptoms, functioning, or quality of life): immediately after the care, when the patient is discharged, or much later?

11. a. Administrative
     b. Clinical
12. change; improvement
13. a. Are the results valid?
     b. What are the results?
     c. How can I apply the results to patient care?

Mixed Methods Research Methodologies

1. b. (quantitative followed by qualitative)
2. b. (quantitative followed by qualitative)
3. a. (quantitative and qualitative at the same time)
4. c. (qualitative followed by quantitative)
5. a. (quantitative and qualitative at the same time)

Outcomes Research Methodologies

1. c
2. e
3. a
4. b
5. d

EXERCISE 3: WEB-BASED INFORMATION AND RESOURCES

Mixed Methods Research

1. https://obssr.od.nih.gov/training/mixed-methods-research/
2. https://pcmh.ahrq.gov/page/mixed-methods-integrating-quantitative-and-qualitative-data-collection-and-analysis-while
3. May be any two of the following:
Use qualitative data to explore quantitative findings.
Develop survey instruments.
Use qualitative data to augment a quantitative outcomes study
Involve community-based stakeholders

Outcomes Research

1. Agency for Healthcare Research and Quality http://www.ahrq.gov/research/index.html
2. American Nurses Association http://www.nursingworld.org/
3. Collaborative Alliance for Nursing Outcomes http://www.calnoc.org/
4. National Database of Nursing Quality Indicators http://www.nursingquality.org/
5. National Institute of Nursing Research http://www.ninr.nih.gov/
6. Nursing Interventions Classification http://www.nursing.uiowa.edu/cncce/nursing-interventions-classification-overview
7. National Quality Forum http://www.qualityforum.org/Home.aspx
8. Oncology Nursing Society http://www.ons.org/Research

EXERCISE 4: CONDUCTING CRITICAL APPRAISALS TO BUILD AN EVIDENCE-BASED PRACTICE

Mixed Methods Research

1. "The purpose of the study was to discover and describe the experiences of total joint replacement patients and their family members who participated in a brief family visit during phase 1 recovery" (Wendler et al., 2017, p. 46).
2. Explanatory sequential
3. a. transferability
   b. confirmability
   c. credibility
   d. dependability
4. "What is the description of what it is like for both patients and family members who experience phase 1 family visits in the PACU?" (Wendler et al., 2017, p. 46).
5. "to see with my own eyes" (Wendler et al., 2017, p. 55).
6. a. W because title should give an indication of the methodology and population.
   b. S because the research team included a nurse with a research-focused doctoral degree and clinical experts.
   c. W because cannot generalize findings from convenience sample from one setting.
   d. S because without a comparison or control group, the participants serving as their own controls was a way to compare pre- and post-levels of anxiety and vital signs.
   e. S because the details about the vital sign monitor increases the reader's confidence that the data that were collected were accurate.
   f. S because the researchers provide evidence that the items on the instrument were reliable.
   g. W if considering that patients and family members may have been influenced by the answers given by the other; S if considering their experience as a joint experience to which they both contributed.
   h. S because connecting study findings to the research framework increases the usefulness of the theory and the nursing knowledge base.

i. W because the study sample was limited to knee replacement patients who received spinal anesthesia. Phase 1 recovery visits may not be safe or appropriate for other surgical patients, especially those who receive general anesthesia.

Outcomes Research

The critical appraisal was of the Dizon, Linos, Arron, Hills, and Chren (2017) study available through an open access journal.

1. The outcome research methodology that was used was secondary analysis. "In this study, we utilized data from a prospective cohort study of all patients with K. C. [keratinocyte carcinomas] diagnosed in 1999–2000...In the parent study, trained nurse practitioners who were blinded to study goals...reviewed all records" (Dizon et al., 2017, p. 2).
2. The clinical process outcomes were cycles of destruction, excisional margins, stages of Mohs surgery, time to treatment, and provision of postoperative pain medication. The clinical outcome was tumor recurrence. The patient-reported outcomes were satisfaction, change in quality of life, cosmetic appearance, and problems encountered (Dizon et al., 2017).
3. "The time to treatment was defined as the number of days between initial biopsy and treatment" (Dizon et al., 2017, p. 2).
4. The sample included 1353 eligible patients with KC. This was a large group of heterogeneous study participants from two types of treatment settings. The sample was appropriate for an outcomes study.
5. The setting for the study was Veterans Affairs clinics and fee-for-service clinics (FFS). No, the participants from the VA were "older, more likely to be male, had lower levels of education, worse self-reported general health, and were most likely to have had a previous history of KC. Tumors treated at the VA were more likely to be treated with excision compared to tumors treated at the FFS." (Dizon et al., 2017, p. 5).
6. a. VA
    b. FFS
    c. VA
7. Can be summarized in your own words, but direct quotation is as follows: "Care for KC in a VA and a FFS practice setting differed in few process measures, but we were unable to detect any substantial or consistent differences in clinical or patient-reported outcomes.... Five-year recurrence rates were equally low in both settings and the majority of patients were satisfied with most domains of care, experienced improvement in skin-related quality of life, rated their cosmetic outcomes favorably, and encountered no problems with care" (Dizon et al., 2017, p. 8–9).
8. Critical appraisal of Dizon et al. (2017) study. The study purpose was clearly stated and appropriate for this outcomes study. The Donabedian Model for quality of care provided the framework for this study and was clearly adapted to care of patients with KC (Figure 1, Dizon et al., 2017, p. 3). The process measures and clinical and patient-reported outcome measures were clearly identified and linked to the study framework. The study design was strong and included data from a prospective cohort study of patients with KC treated in either a FFS dermatology practice or a VA dermatology practice. The sample size was large with 1353 patients who had varied backgrounds and were recruited from different settings (FFS and VA clinics). The analytic strategies were clearly described and appropriate for this outcomes study.

    The researchers identified limitations related to the sample and measurement strategies that decreased the generalization of the study findings. The study conclusion was consistent with the results and findings and indicated: "Quality of ambulatory surgical care for KC, assessed by both clinical and patient-reported measures, was similar in government-operated managed care practice and a fee-for-service practice" (Dizon et al., 2017, p. 9-10). This study fills a gap in the knowledge about care for the most common skin cancers in ambulatory settings.

Donna Hallas, Mary Koslap-Petraco and Jason Fletcher Study

Journal of Pediatric Nursing 33 (2017) 33–40

Contents lists available at ScienceDirect

Journal of Pediatric Nursing

ELSEVIER

Social-Emotional Development of Toddlers: Randomized Controlled Trial of an Office-Based Intervention

 CrossMark

Donna Hallas [a,*], Mary Koslap-Petraco [b,c], Jason Fletcher [a]

[a] New York University Rory Meyers College of Nursing, New York, NY, United States
[b] Long Island University Post, Brookville, NY, United States
[c] Suffolk County Department of Health, Coordinator Child Health, Great River, NY, United States

ARTICLE INFO

Article history:
Received 27 April 2016
Revised 1 November 2016
Accepted 20 November 2016

Keywords:
Toddler
Social-emotional development
Maternal confidence

ABSTRACT

Purpose: During the toddler years, temper tantrums and impulsive behaviors are the norm. These behaviors can frustrate even the most experienced mothers.
Design and Methods: A prospective, double blind, randomized controlled trial using pre-test/post-test experimental design was used to examine the effectiveness of an office-based educational program to improve maternal confidence and the social-emotional development of toddlers. The Toddler Care Questionnaire (TCQ) was administered to all mothers as a pre and post intervention test. The treatment intervention was a videotaped (DVD) parenting skills intervention on the social-emotional development of toddlers and on maternal confidence in caring for toddlers.
Results: Sixty mothers and 60 toddlers entered the study with 29 mothertoddler dyads randomized to the treatment group and 31 to the control group. Twenty-six (26) mother-toddler dyads in the treatment and 25 mother-toddler dyads in the control group completed the study. Pairwise comparisons of adjusted means showed significant improvements for both toddler groups on the Brigance toddler screen, and no statistically significant difference in gains between the groups. The mixed model results for the TCQ showed an overall significant improvement from preto post-test, and a non-significant interaction between group and time indicting no significant difference in gains seen by treatment groups.
Conclusions: Brief educational programs on DVD's are an efficient way to offer information to mothers while in the office waiting area. Practice Implications: Pediatric nurses who encounter mothers who struggle with caring for their toddlers may find brief-office based interventions a valuable tool for educating parents.
© 2016 Elsevier Inc. All rights reserved.

Introduction

Background

Today toddlers are being raised in a variety of traditional and complex family situations. During the toddler years, temper tantrums and impulsive behaviors are the norm. These behaviors can frustrate even the most experienced mothers. This frustration is evident in the 2014 national data that show the youngest children are the most vulnerable: 27% of the reported victims of child abuse and neglect are under the age of three (Center for Disease Control and Prevention (CDC) Injury prevention and Control Division of Violence Prevention, 2016). Children's Bureau An Office of the Administration for Children and Families (2014) (https://www.childwelfare.gov/pubPDFs/fatality.pdf)

reported that an estimated 1580 children died from child abuse and neglect, representing a rate of four children dying every day in the U.S. from abuse and neglect. Children under the age of three accounted for 70.7% of these fatalities: 40.1% were infants and 33.6% were between one and three years old (https://www.childwelfare.gov/pubPDFs/fatality.pdf).

Lerner and Ciervo (2010) conducted a public opinion poll by interviewing 1615 parents of children ages birth to 36 months. The authors reported that parents of toddlers confront the following behaviors on a regular basis: temper tantrums, crying and controlling emotions, biting and fighting, not listening, sleeping and bedtime issues, potty training, and food issues (Lerner & Ciervo). Toddler behaviors viewed as problematic by mothers have been linked to maternal negative behaviors and stress (Calkins, 2002). Adverse toddler behaviors have been identified as a precursor to low maternal self-esteem and a lack of maternal confidence (Hutchings, Appleton, Smith, Lane, & Nash, 2002). Walker and Sprague (2000) concluded that once social-emotional problems are established in a young child, it is difficult to

* Corresponding author: Donna Hallas.
  E-mail addresses: dh88@nyu.edu (D. Hallas), Mary.Koslap-Petraco@liu.edu (M. Koslap-Petraco), Fletcj01@nyu.edu (J. Fletcher).

http://dx.doi.org/10.1016/j.pedn.2016.11.004
0882-5963/© 2016 Elsevier Inc. All rights reserved.

34 *D. Hallas et al. / Journal of Pediatric Nursing 33 (2017) 33–40*

alter their behavior, as the children are highly resistant to change. Other researchers have confirmed that untreated social-emotional problems become chronic problems as the child continues to age (Cooper, Masi, & Vick, 2009; DelCarmen-Wiggins & Carter, 2001; Zimmer-Gembeck et al., 2015). The prevalence of social-emotional problems among toddlers has been estimated to be between 9.5% and 14.2% of children between birth and 5-years old (Brauner & Stephens, 2006). The prevalence of social-emotional problems for children living in at-risk environments is estimated to be between 17% and 25% and the children are more likely to have behavioral problems that adversely impact their development (Knapp, Ammen, Arstein-Kerslake, Poulsen, & Mastergeorge, 2007).

Positive maternal-toddler interactions high in maternal sensitivity to the needs of the toddler have been linked to positive outcomes for the toddler and include a more secure mother-toddler attachment (Ainsworth, Blehar, Waters, & Wall, 1978; Clucas, Skar, Sherr, & von Tetzchner, 2014; DeWolff & van Ijzendoorn, 1997) and fewer behavioral problems exhibited by the toddler (Smith, Calkins, Keane, Anastopoulos, & Shelton, 2004). Sugisawa et al. (2010) examined the trajectory patterns of parenting by caregivers raising toddlers and its effect on the social competence of the toddlers. The researchers used the Interaction Rating Scale (IRS) to evaluate toddler social competence and the Index of Child Care Environment (ICCE) to analyze the caregivers' responses to the toddler. Sugisawa et al. concluded that the development of toddler social competence is directly related to consistent and positive parenting.

Researchers have demonstrated that parenting programs focusing on behavioral changes can have a positive short-term effect on the mother's psychosocial health (Barlow, Coren, & Stewart-Brown, 2003). Mendelsohn et al. (2007) conducted a randomized controlled trial (RCT) using videotaped interactions by child developmental specialists for 99 Latina mothers to support toddler development. The results revealed decreased levels of parenting stress, an increase in cognitive development and decrease in developmental delays displayed by the toddlers in the treatment group. The researchers concluded that pediatric primary care-based interventions can effectively improve development in toddlers. Hayes, Matthew, Copley, and Welsh (2007) conducted a RCT of a mother-toddler parenting program and demonstrated that delivery of a one-day intervention for distressed mothers contributed to reducing parental stress and an improvement in reducing toddler behavior problems.

Olds, Sadler, and Kitzman (2007) conducted a review of the evidence from 19 RCT's that focused on promoting parenting of infants and toddlers prior to the emergence of parenting problems. The researchers discussed the importance of following the Institute of Medicine's rigor for design and implementation of RCTs using the principles of epidemiology and theory. They also recommended conducting smaller trials to assure the success of the intervention before conducting large scale RCTs. Olds et al., concluded that programs in which visiting nurses began parenting interventions with high-risk families during the prenatal period and with first time mothers during the infant's first two years of life were most successful in improving the prenatal health of the mother and subsequently the child's health and development when the nurses were specifically trained to provide services to the parents.

Buss and Kiel (2010) examined changes over time of toddlers' fearful behaviors when protective mothering behaviors were employed. They found that maternal protective behaviors were directly related to regulation of their toddlers' distress. They concluded that their study contributes initial evidence that in-the-moment influence between parents and toddlers is important for control of the toddlers' fearful behaviors.

The impetus for conducting our RCT were general observations made by the Principal Investigator (PI) and Co-Investigator (Co-I) of mother-toddler interactions in waiting areas in a pediatric primary care office in which mothers were interacting inappropriately with toddlers escalating challenging toddler behaviors. The mother-toddler interactions were also viewed as impeding the social-emotional development of these toddlers. Thus, an urgency to implement strategies to improve mother-toddler interactions, the social-emotional development of toddlers, and potentially reduce the potential for harm to toddlers was the rationale for the study design.

The focus of this study was to evaluate the effectiveness of a pediatric primary care office-based parenting skills intervention to improve 1) maternal confidence in caring for a toddler and 2) the social-emotional development of toddlers.

Theoretical and Evidence-Based Development of the Treatment Intervention

The treatment interventions, designed by the PI and Co-I, were based on Watson's caring theoretical framework, specifically the helping-trusting relationship (Watson, 1997, 2003). At the center of the helping-trusting relationship is the intercommunication and transpersonal identity with the concomitant release of human feelings for each other (Watson, 1997). A helping and trusting relationship evolves in caring moments when the mother embraces the toddler in times of opposing emotions such as love/anger, happiness/frustration, and is accepting of both the positive and negative feelings expressed by the toddler.

For teenage mothers to develop a helping-trusting relationship with their toddler, they need to meet their own adolescent developmental milestones as they progress through the turbulent teenage years with the goal of growing into successful adults. Adolescent parenting is an early transition to an adult role that is out of sequence with the social norms of the adolescent (Jemmott, Jemmott, Hutchinson, Cederbaum, & O'Leary, 2008). A high level of teen parental stress is expected. Parental stress has been shown to have a direct negative effect on the psychological health of young children of teenage mothers (Cooper et al., 2009). However, parental stress and toddler behaviors can adversely affect the maternal confidence of all mothers caring for toddlers, with a resultant decrease in the social-emotional development of toddlers (Cooper et al.) The premise for the treatment intervention is based on evidence that mothers of all ages who are actively involved in the process of physically and emotionally caring for the toddler and who are sensitive and affectionate towards the toddler in their daily interactions will experience personal 'growth in connection' (Surrey, 1991) to the toddler and foster the development of maternal confidence. The feelings of 'connectedness' of the mother to the toddler that emerges from mutual feelings of caring were hypothesized to increase the social-emotional development of the toddler (Hallas, 2002).

Objectives

The objectives for this RCT were to evaluate the impact of a pediatric primary care office-based videotaped (DVD) parenting skills intervention on 1) the social-emotional development of toddlers and 2) maternal confidence for mothers raising toddlers.

Hypothesis

1. There will be a greater increase in the social-emotional development of toddlers as measured by the Brigance Toddler Screen for toddlers whose mothers receive the treatment intervention (treatment group) in a pediatric primary care office-based practice as compared to toddlers in the control group whose mothers receive the standard office-based care.
2. There will be a greater increase in maternal confidence for mothers who receive the parenting skills intervention (treatment group) in a pediatric primary care office-based practice as measured by the Toddler Care Questionnaire (TCQ) compared to mothers in the control group who receive the standard office-based care.

D. Hallas et al. / Journal of Pediatric Nursing 33 (2017) 33–40   35

Methods

Trial Design

A prospective, double blind, randomized controlled trial using pre-test/post-test experimental design was used to test the effectiveness of a videotaped (DVD) parenting skills intervention on the social-emotional development of toddlers and on maternal confidence of mothers caring for their toddlers.

Institutional Review Board

Institutional Review Board (IRB) approval was obtained to conduct the study from New York University, Washington Square. Following this approval, SCO Family of Services and New York State Department of Health, and Suffolk County Department of Health and Mental Health Services provided IRB approval to conduct the study in their clinics. The physician who owned the private practice reviewed the study and the New York University IRB approval and then consented to have the study conducted in his office.

Participants

The target populations were mother-toddler dyads in which the mother was interacting with and raising the toddler in any of the following family structures: two-parent, single parent, extended family members, group homes for teen mothers between the ages of 15 to 19-years old, first time and experienced mothers, grandmothers who were the primary caretakers of the toddlers, and foster care mothers.

Inclusion Criteria

All mothers, who spoke English or Spanish, who were responsible for caring for a toddler who received their primary healthcare in one of the participating pediatric offices, were eligible to participate in the study.

All toddlers who were between the ages of 12 to 33 months at the start of the study and came for a primary health care visit with their mother met inclusion criteria as a mother-toddler dyad participant.

Exclusion Criteria

All mothers of toddlers who could not speak or understand English or Spanish were excluded from the study. All mothers of toddlers who refused to sign informed consent were excluded from the study. If a toddler refused to participate in assessment activities on the Brigance Toddler screen, this behavior would be considered refusal of toddler assent per IRB study approval, and the toddler and mother were excluded as study participants. Biological parents for children in foster care were excluded from this study, as they were not providing the day-to-day care for the toddler during the study period.

Study Settings

Five pediatric primary healthcare offices participated as study sites and included offices and clinics in Brooklyn, Queens, Manhattan, and Suffolk County, New York. Each office provided comprehensive primary health care to children who resided in borough or County. The children in the study were insured through private insurers, Child Health Plus, a NY State health insurance plan for lower income children, Medicaid managed care, or were uninsured or underinsured (New York State Department of Health Child Health Plus web site, 1985). The offices and clinic populations matched the general demographics of the boroughs and county, however our study sample differed in Queens and Brooklyn with a greater representation of Whites and Latinos than reported populations in these two boroughs. Primary care services were provided to the children by pediatric nurse practitioners, pediatricians, registered nurses and licensed practical nurses.

Interventions

Treatment Intervention

Two-treatment intervention DVDs were designed: One for teenage mothers and one for all other mothers. The only difference between the teenage mother intervention DVD and the treatment intervention DVD for all other mothers was an additional one-minute discussion on being a teenage mother. Teenage development in comparison to toddler development was discussed. Feelings of conflict between the teenager and the toddler were discussed and strategies to aid the teen to believe that teenagers are capable mothers by viewing their strengths before their problems was described through examples. All other intervention strategies were identical (Table 1).

The treatment DVD presentation focused on the joy of "caring for" the "Terrific Toddler" (Hallas & Koslap-Petraco, 2007) which represents a paradigm shift from the worldview of the "Terrible Two's" and is consistent with Watson's theory of caring (Watson, 1997) and growth in connection (Surrey, 1991) and connectedness (Hallas, 2002; Hallas & Koslap-Petraco, 2004). The DVD was available in English and Spanish.

Control Intervention

The control group intervention was a standardized DVD on toddler nutrition (Parents Action for Children, 2006). The DVD was available in English and Spanish. The wrapping for the DVD was the same as the one for the intervention DVD, thus the identification of the DVD contents (treatment and control) were concealed from the mothers, the RNs and research assistants (RAs).

Procedures

Prior to recruiting subjects, the PI and Co-I met with the physicians, NPs, RNs, and office staff at each site and trained the RNs and RAs on study recruitment process, subject eligibility, study interventions, and process for obtaining informed consent. Fliers were then posted in each practice site that agreed to permit the researchers to recruit and invite all mothers, eligible by inclusion criteria, and their respective toddlers to participate in the study. Each mother who volunteered to participate in the study provided written informed consent prior to enrollment in the study. After enrollment, each mother-toddler dyad was given a folder that had been randomized into either the treatment or control group using a computer-generated random numbers list created by the study biostatistician. All RNs and RAs were blinded to folder contents, as all folders were identical and the DVDs were all labeled with a code only known to the PI. The folders with the pre-test results were given to the PI and all participants identifying information was removed from the folder to assure anonymity. Each folder only contained the randomized number for the participant dyads. The names of the

Table 1
Outline for the contents of the DVD office-based treatment intervention.

Toddler growth and developmental norms
Developing the helping trusting relationship: "The Terrific Two's"
   Communicating with toddlers: Understanding the meaning of 'No"
   Talking calmly
   Consistent maternal responses to the toddler needs
Playing with the toddler to improve social-emotional development
Understanding Challenging toddler behaviors
   Impulsivity: definition and how to manage
   Temper Tantrums: definition and how to manage
   Hugging the toddler during times of stress: Improving Toddler coping skills
Information included for Teenage Mothers: Building the Relationship
   Recognition of teenage maternal strengths
   Comparison of Teen feelings to Toddler emotions and behaviors
    Impulsivity and control of feelings of anger and frustration

Interventions designed by the PI and Co-I based on best available evidence.

36   *D. Hallas et al. / Journal of Pediatric Nursing 33 (2017) 33–40*

participants and their randomized numbers were maintained in a separate secured filed cabinet in the office of the PI. Data were collected from June 30, 2009 to September 30, 2010. There were no changes to the IRB approved trial design before or during data collection.

Outcome Assessments: Toddler Care Questionnaire and Brigance Toddler Screen

Instrument #1

The Toddler Care Questionnaire (TCQ) (Gross & Rocissano, 1988, 1989) is a measure of maternal confidence for all mothers of toddlers between the ages of 12 and 36 months (Table 2). Thirty-seven item responses are scored from A to E and equated to the numbers 1 to 5. The range in total scores is from 37 to 185. Higher scores reflect greater maternal confidence. The TCQ instrument reliability is reported to be between 0.91 and 0.96 and test-retest reliability is 0.87. Office personnel gave the TCQ to the mothers to complete while in the office waiting area prior to the child's visit. The responses from the mothers on both the pretest and posttest for each TCQ were placed in the mother's respective folder and given to the PI to enter data in SPSS for the statistical analysis (IBM Corp. Released 2013. IBM SPSS Statistics for Windows, Version 22.0. Armonk, NY: IBM Corp.).

Instrument #2

The Brigance Toddler Screen (Brigance & Glascoe, 2002) was used for toddlers between the ages of 12 to 33 months old (Table 3). The Brigance screens for social-emotional skills and consists of 10 items. One point is given for each item the toddler is able to perform with a total score of 10 points possible. Higher scores are indicative of higher social-emotional development. Test-retest reliability for the Brigance Toddler Screen is reported at 0.98 to 0.99. Specificity for the Brigance toddler screen was reported as ranging from 85% to 86% and sensitivity ranged from 76% to 77%. The RN or RA in the respective primary care office administered the Brigance screen. The Brigance toddler screen was completed in approximately 1 min.

Sample Size

A priori power analysis was conducted for each outcome to ascertain the sample size necessary to attain a power of 0.80 with a type I error rate of 0.05 for the minimally relevant effect using independent groups *t*-tests (Baker Bausell & Li, 2002). Estimates of variability from the literature were used in calculations. Theses analyses indicated a sample size of 30 mothers and toddlers for each group would provide sufficient power to detect the estimated effect.

Randomization: Sequence Generation and Type

For allocation of participants, the biostatistician created a computer generated list of random numbers. The PI labeled files in each of the offices using the computer generated list to randomly assign participants to either the treatment or control group.

Randomization: Allocation Concealment Mechanism

The allocation sequence was concealed from the RNs and RAs enrolling and assessing participants at each study site. The files containing the TCQ and Brigance questionnaires were the same. The only difference was the randomized number that did not have any meaning to the RNs or RAs. The signed consent form was placed in the file and only the PI created a list of participant names and linked them to the randomized numbers. The consent form was then separated from the file and the PI made a separate list of names of participants from each study site. All participants completed the same study instruments, thus no information about the group assignment was known to the RNs or RAs. Since all participants watched a DVD privately, the participants did not know if they were assigned to the treatment or control group (Table 4).

Table 2
Toddler care questionnaire (TCQ).

1. Knowing which toys are appropriate for your child's age
2. Knowing how to encourage your child's language development
3. Knowing about common fears child have at this age
4. Knowing what to do to help your child develop hand coordination (for example using a spoon; stacking blocks)
5. Knowing how to help your child develop body coordination (for example; walking and climbing)
6. Knowing how to manage toilet training
7. Knowing how feeding patterns change between 12 and 36 months
8. Knowing which situations are likely to upset your child
9. Knowing how to make your home safe for your child
10. Knowing which situation your child is likely to enjoy
11. Predicting how your child will respond to new people and places
12. Knowing your child's daily sleep schedule
13. Knowing what foods your child will or will not eat
14. Predicting whether your child will like a new toy
15. Knowing what your child's different cries mean (for example tiredness, hunger, pain, fear, boredom, frustration)
16. Knowing how to relieve your child's distress (for example, due to being tired, hungry, in pain, frightened, bored, frustrated)
17. Involving your child in activities you both enjoy
18. Knowing when your child seems to want affection from you
19. Being comfortable in showing affection to your child
20. Getting your child to smile or laugh
21. Getting your child to calm down when upset
22. Know your child's favorite games and toys
23. Knowing how to help your child play with other children
24. Helping your child adjust to new situations (for example a new babysitter, entering daycare, vacationing, etc.)
25. Setting limits on your child's destructive behaviors (for example, tearing books, breaking valuable items)
26. Setting limits on your child's behavior when it looks dangerous (for example playing with electric outlets and wires)
27. Knowing hate types of discipline does not work with your child
28. Knowing what to do when your child has a temper tantrum
29. Getting your child to bed without a problem
30. Keeping a consistent bedtime hour for your child
31. Knowing when rules can be "bent" or modified and when they should not be
32. Getting back to "friendly terms" with your child soon after a problem behavior has ended
33. Knowing whether your style of parenting will "spoil" a child
34. Managing your child's aggressiveness with other children (for example, hitting pushing, biting)
35. Finding supportive services in your community for you and your child (for example, other parents of young children, play groups)
36. Knowing how to manage non-emergency illnesses at home (for example, fever, diarrhea, minor injuries)
37. Managing separations from your child (for example, to go to the store, to go to work, to go out for the evening)

Gross and Rocissano (1988).

Table 3
Brigance toddler screen.

Activity	Performs		Yes	No	Score
1. Play pat-a-cake	Yes	No			
2. Shows affection	Yes	No			
3. Shows an interest in others	Yes	No			
4. Imitates interactions	Yes	No			
5. Shows pride and pleasure	Yes	No			
6. Explores and returns	Yes	No			
7. Imitates other children	Yes	No			
8. Watches faces for clues	Yes	No			
9. Mimics adult activities	Yes	No			
10. Performs for others	Yes	No			

Scores 1 point for each activity the toddler can perform.
Brigance and Glascoe (2002).

D. Hallas et al. / Journal of Pediatric Nursing 33 (2017) 33–40

Table 4
Participants.

Social-Emotional Development of Toddlers: Randomized Controlled Trial of an Office-Based Intervention

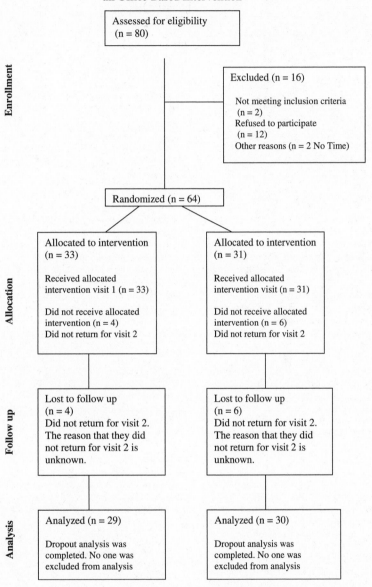

Dropout

Thirty-three mother-toddler dyads were randomized to enter the treatment group and 31 mother-toddler dyads were randomized to enter the control group. Twenty-nine mother-toddler dyads in the treatment group and 30 mother-toddler dyads in the control group completed the initial visit. A total of 26 mother-toddler dyads from the treatment group and 25 mother-toddler dyads from the control group completed the follow-up visit. All mothers were called to return for the routine health care appointments, as per the policies of the various offices. A total of 9 mothers did not return to complete the second visit. Reasons why the mothers did not return were not known. The results for dropout analysis are in Table 5.

Data Analysis

The primary outcomes were pre- and post-test scores for mothers' maternal confidence as measured by TCQ, and toddlers' social-emotional development as measured by the Brigance toddler screen during the 3-month study timeframe.

The adequacy of randomization and impact of dropout was assessed by comparing groups defined by treatment arm and study completion status on demographic and baseline study variables. Comparisons were made using Fisher's exact test for categorical variables and independent groups t-tests for continuous variables. These preliminary analyses indicated that mothers who completed the study had significantly higher mean baseline TCQ scores compared to those that did not return

38   *D. Hallas et al. / Journal of Pediatric Nursing 33 (2017) 33–40*

Table 5
Comparison of dyads by completion status.

	Dropout (*n* = 9)		Complete (*n* = 51)		
	n	%	n	%	*p*
Treatment group					0.474[†]
Treatment	3	10.3	26	89.7	
Control	6	19.4	25	80.6	
Race/Ethnicity					0.482[†]
Hispanic	5	19.2	21	80.8	
Non-Hispanic	4	11.8	30	88.2	
Occasional help from babysitter	8	100.0	44	86.3	0.578[†]
Toddler goes to day care	4	50.0	14	27.5	0.231[†]
Other children in the home	2	25.0	21	41.2	0.464[†]
Mother works full- or part-time	3	37.5	15	29.4	0.690[†]
	M	SD	M	SD	*p*
Mother's age (years)	31.3	4.8	31.1	12.3	0.950[‡]
Baby's age (months)	20.6	8.9	18.3	5.9	0.352[‡]
Baseline TCQ	133.8	22.5	152.9	24.5	0.042[‡]
Baseline Brigance	1.9	2.3	7.9	1.8	0.970[‡]

[†] Fisher's exact test.
[‡] Independent groups *t*-test.

Table 6
Participant characteristics and pretest baseline scores.

	Treatment		Control		
	n	%	n	%	*p*
Completed study (% of randomized)	26	78.8	25	78.1	1.0[†]
Race/Ethnicity					0.60[†]
Latina	14	53.8	11	44.0	
Black	6	23.1	8	32.0	
White	2	7.7	4	16.0	
Other	4	15.4	2	8.0	
Occasional help from babysitter	28	96.6	24	80.0	0.103[†]
Toddler goes to day care	6	20.7	12	40.0	0.158[†]
Other children in the home	10	34.5	13	43.3	0.596[†]
Mother works full- or part-time	6	20.7	12	40.0	0.158[†]
	M	SD	M	SD	*p*
Mother's age (years)	28	10.2	34.1	12.1	0.042[‡]
Baby's age (months)	20.2	7.2	17.3	5.2	0.096[‡]
Baseline TCQ	152.2	25.5	148.6	24.7	0.583[‡]
Baseline Brigance	8.1	1.8	7.7	1.9	0.410[‡]

[†] Fisher's exact test.
[‡] Independent groups *t*-test.

for post-test. In light of this, mixed regression models were conducted following an intent to treat (ITT) strategy to examine change over time in outcomes measures (TCQ and Brigance). Unlike "complete case" methods for analyzing change over time (e.g. RMANOVA) that exclude data from individuals with incomplete records, mixed models are able to incorporate all available data. In the presence of incomplete data (e.g. missing follow up) baseline observations are still used in the estimation of treatment effects, reducing the potential for bias in the estimation of treatment effects. The models included fixed effects for treatment group, time (pre/post) and an interaction term (group by time) to assess whether gains differed between treatment groups. Random effects were used to incorporate for individual variability in the model. Maternal age differed between treatment groups, and so was included in regression models as a covariate. Bonferroni-corrected comparisons were conducted to evaluate group-level change in adjusted mean scores over time. A two-tailed significance level of 0.05 was used for all statistical analyses. Analyses were performed with SPSS (IBM Corp. Released 2013. IBM SPSS Statistics for Windows, Version 22.0. Armonk, NY: IBM Corp.).

Results

Mothers who participated in this study were between the ages of 17 to 62 years old: with the average age of 28.0 years in the treatment group (age range 18 to 62 years) and average age range of 34.1 years in the control group (age range 17 to 60 years). The toddlers ranged in age from 8 to 33 months old at the start of the study. A total of 60 mothers and 60 toddlers entered the study with 29 mother-toddler dyads randomized to the treatment group and 31 to the control group. Twenty-six (26) mother-toddler dyads in the treatment and 25 mother-toddler dyads in the control group completed the study. Completion rates did not differ significantly between treatment groups.

There were no significant differences between dyads who completed the study and those who completed only the baseline visit in terms of ethnicity, use of day care, other children in the home, maternal employment, mother's and baby's ages or baseline Brigance scores (Table 5). Mothers who only completed baseline did report significantly lower levels of maternal confidence ($t(57) = 2.08, p = 0.042$). Mothers in the treatment and control groups were similar in completion rates, ethnicity, day care use, other children in the home, maternal employment, baby's age, and baseline TCQ and Brigance scores (Table 6). Mothers in the treatment group were significantly younger than mothers in the control group ($t(57) = 2.079, p = 0.042$) (Table 6).

Overall, mother-toddler dyads in both treatment and control groups showed an increase on both the TCQ (Fig. 1) and the Brigance (Fig. 2).

The mixed model results for the TCQ showed an overall significant improvement from pre- to post-test, and a non-significant interaction between group and time indicting no significant difference in gains seen by treatment groups. Bonferroni-corrected multiple comparisons of adjusted means indicated that while both groups improved, only the treatment group improved significantly ($p = 0.002$) (Table 7). Gains seen by the intervention group were nearly twice as large as that seen for the control group. Despite the large difference in improvement between the two groups, the interaction term was non-significant, likely due to the limited statistical power in the small sample size.

Both the intervention and control groups of toddlers showed a significant improvement in social-emotional development as measured by the Brigance toddler screen, gaining >1 point (Control 1.1, $p = 0.001$ and Intervention 1.4, $p < 0.001$) (adjusted means and confidence intervals presented in Table 8). There was a significant effect for time, but the interaction between group and time was non-significant showing no significant differences in gains between the intervention and control group.

Discussion

A primary care pediatric office-based educational intervention was designed to improve maternal confidence while raising toddlers and to improve the social-emotional development of toddlers. The study

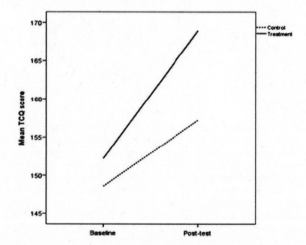

Fig. 1. Baseline and posttest scores TCQ.

D. Hallas et al. / Journal of Pediatric Nursing 33 (2017) 33–40   39

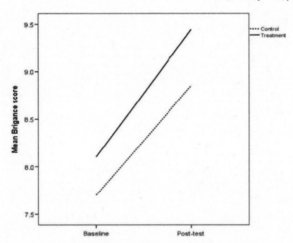

Fig. 2. Baseline and posttest scores Brigance.

Table 8
Brigance pretest and posttest analysis.

Brigance						
	Pre			Post		
Treatment group	M	CI 95%		M	CI 95%		*p*
Intervention	8	7.4	8.6	9.4	8.7	9.9	<0.001
Control	7.8	7.2	8.4	8.9	8.3	9.6	0.001

design was a prospective, double blind, randomized controlled trial using a pre-test post-test experimental design to determine the effectiveness of the intervention.

Hypothesis one was not supported. Toddlers in both the treatment and control groups improved in their performance on the Brigance toddler screen over the 3-month study period. While we did not find significant differences between treatment groups, the fact that all toddlers improved is notable as the majority of the participants were from high-risk social environments. Our findings of improvement over time cannot be directly related to our study interventions, however, the interventions fostered basic parenting skills that have the potential to improve toddler social-emotional development over time. Fuller, Bein, Kim, and Rabe-Hesketh (2015) report findings from their research on early growth and the relationship on the levels of cognitive and communication skills of Mexican American and native born White mothers at 9 and 24 months of age. They concluded that the educational background of the mother and parenting practices were positively correlated to the growth of the toddler over the 9 to 24-month period. The children showed the most cognitive development when the mothers had some college education, and engaged in daily reading and storytelling with their toddlers.

The second hypothesis was supported. The results showed a significant difference for the treatment group of mother-toddler dyads in the mothers' maternal confidence in caring for toddlers as measured by the TCQ. The statistically significant improvement in maternal confidence for mothers in the treatment group is an important outcome. Pediatric primary care providers who encounter mothers on a daily basis who struggle with caring for their impetuous toddlers may find brief-office based interventions a valuable tool for educating parents not only to improve maternal confidence for raising toddlers, but also to educate the mothers on specific growth and development patterns. Our study results are consistent with a recent study of 89 toddlers and their mothers who were from economically vulnerable homes in which the mothers were educated about emotion talk with their toddlers (Brophy-Herb et al., 2015). The researchers concluded that the highest risk toddlers benefited the most from the mother's emotion talk with the toddlers.

The dropout analysis revealed that mothers who only completed baseline testing and visit 1 had significantly lower maternal confidence scores than mothers in both the treatment and control groups who completed both visits. We cannot predict the study outcomes for these dropout mothers, but what our clinical experiences as pediatric nurse practitioners have revealed that mothers who are frequent 'no shows' for scheduled primary care office visits for their children are those who are most in-need of parent education to support the normal growth and development of their children.

Brief office-based educational programs on DVD's are an easy, cost-effective, effective, and efficient way to offer educational programs to mothers while in the waiting areas for a well child visit. Future studies or a replication of this study with a larger sample size are needed to add to the body of knowledge on the relationship between maternal confidence and improving the social-emotional development of toddlers.

Implications for Pediatric RN's and Nurse Practitioners

During the many years of experience in primary care settings, the PI and Co-I had seen first-hand the difficulty parents experience while raising toddlers. They also recognized the adverse effect on toddler behaviors when parents reacted negatively to what were viewed developmentally by the PNPs as normal toddler behaviors. The investigators believed that the social-emotional development of toddlers could be strengthened if mothers were educated during primary care office visits to better understand typical toddler behaviors. Empowering mothers by increasing their confidence in parenting their toddlers is relevant to pediatric nursing care for toddlers.

Pediatric nurses and nurse practitioners in primary care settings have a unique opportunity and yet a small window of time to help mothers of toddlers learns about successful parenting behaviors. Thus, a brief office-based DVD educational intervention designed for mothers to view in waiting areas prior to the routine office visit is an easy format to use and was acceptable and welcoming by the mothers in our study. During the office visit, the pediatric nurse or NP can ask if the mother has any questions about the DVD content and then focus on a particular problem that the mother may acknowledge during the visit. When mothers are taught how to understand the behaviors of their toddlers, they may feel empowered to respond positively to the toddler, improving both their personal feelings about parenting and the social-emotional development of their toddlers. Pediatric nurses and nurse practitioners are encouraged to replicate this study in primary care offices to provide the same level of care for mother-toddler dyads and to share their outcomes on changes in maternal confidence and toddler social-emotional development. Doctoral of Nursing Practice (DNP) graduates and/or students may to consider implementing a quality improvement study using this educational intervention to determine the effect on maternal confidence and toddler social-emotional development.

Limitations of the Study

The generalizability of this study is limited due to the small sample size that limited the statistical power of this study. Replication of this study using a larger study sample may be beneficial as there are few

Table 7
TCQ pretest and posttest analysis.

	TCQ						
	Pre			Post			
Treatment group	M	CI 95%		M	CI 95%		*p*
Intervention	152.9	144.3	161.5	169.7	160.6	178.7	0.002
Control	147.9	139.4	156.4	156.5	147.3	165.7	0.103

rigorously conducted RCTs investigating the social-emotional development of toddlers.

While we followed a rigorous approach for randomization of study participants, mothers in the treatment group were significantly younger than those in the control group which may have affected the level of confidence of the mothers prior to the treatment based on maternal age. Even though we used five different primary care settings within culturally diverse populations, we had a greater representation of white and Latino families in some of the practice settings, therefore, African American families may have been underrepresented.

Conflicts of Interest

None.

Acknowledgements

The authors would like to acknowledge the following:

Greta Westman BS, RN
New York University College of Nursing
Undergraduate Research Assistant
Melissa Mueller BS, RN
New York University College of Nursing
Undergraduate Research Assistant
Rajit Iftikhar
Research Assistant
Suffolk County Department of Health Services
Hauppaugue, New York
SCO Family of Services permitting data collection at two sites
Suffolk County Department of Health for permitting data collection
All authors:

This study received funding from a competitive grant application to New York University Research Fund. The funding source had no involvement in study design, data collection, or data analysis and interpretation of data; in the writing of the report; and in the decision to submit the manuscript for publication.

References

Ainsworth, M. D., Blehar, M. C., Waters, E., & Wall, S. (1978). *Patterns of attachment: A psychological study of strange situation.* Hillsdale, N.J: Erlbaum.

Baker Bausell, R., & Li, Y. -F. (2002). *Power analysis for experimental research: A practical guide for the biological, medical, and social sciences.* Cambridge, NY: Cambridge University Press.

Barlow, J., Coren, E., & Stewart-Brown, S. S. (2003). Parent training programmes for improving maternal psychosocial health. *Cochrane Databased of Systematic Reviews*(Issue 4). http://dx.doi.org/10.1002/14651858.CD002020.pub2 http://www2.cochrane.org/reviews/en/ab002020.html (Art. No.: CD002020).

Brauner, C. B., & Stephens, B. C. (2006). Estimating the prevalence of early childhood serious emotional/behavioral disorder: Challenges and recommendations. *Public Health Reports, 121,* 303–310.

Brigance, A., & Glascoe, F. P. (2002). *Brigance infant toddler screen.* North Billencia, MA: Curriculum Associates, Inc.

Brophy-Herb, H. E., Bocknek, E. L., Vallotton, C. D., Stansbury, K. E., Senehi, N., Dalimonte-Mercking, D., & Lee, Y. (2015). Toddlers with early behavioral problems at higher family demographic risk benefit the most from maternal emotion talk. *Journal of Developmental and Behavioral Pediatrics, 36,* 512–520.

Buss, K. A., & Kiel, E. J. (2010). Maternal accuracy and behavior in anticipating children responses to novelty: Relations to fearful temperament and implications for anxiety development. *Social development, 19,* 304–325.

Calkins, S. D. (2002). Does aversive behavior during toddlerhood matter? The effects of difficult temperament on material perceptions and behavior. *Infant Mental Health Journal, 23,* 381–402.

Center for Disease Control and Prevention (CDC) Injury prevention and Control Division of Violence Prevention (2016). *Child abuse and neglect prevention.* www.cdc.gov (Page last updated May 25, 2016).

Children's Bureau An Office of the Administration for Children (2014). *Child maltreatment reports 2014 Content and Excel tables.* Retrieved from www.acf.hhs.gov/cb/research-data-technology/statistics-reserach/child-maltreatment.

Clucas, C., Skar, A. S., Sherr, L., & von Tetzchner, S. (2014). Mothers and fathers attending the international child development programme in Norway. *The Family Journal: Counseling and Therapy for Couples and Families, 22,* 409–418.

Cooper, J. L., Masi, R., & Vick, J. (2009). *Social-emotional development in early childhood: What every policymaker should know. National Center for Children in.* Poverty: Columbia University, Mailman School of Public Health, Department of Health Policy and Management http://www.nccp.org/publications/pub_882.html.

DelCarmen-Wiggins, R., & Carter, A. S. (2001). Assessment of infant and toddler mental health: Advances and challenges. *Journal of the American Academy of Child and Adolescent Psychiatry, 40,* 8–10.

DeWolff, M. S., & van Ijzendoorn, M. H. (1997). Sensitivity and attachment: A meta-analysis on parental antecedents of infant attachment. *Child Development, 68,* 571–591.

Fuller, B., Bein, E., Kim, Y., & Rabe-Hesketh, S. (2015). Differing cognitive trajectories of Mexican American toddlers: The role of class, nativity, and maternal practices. *Hispanic Journal of Behavioral Sciences, 37,* 139–169.

Gross, D., & Rocissano, L. (1988). Maternal confidence in toddlerhood: A measurement for clinical practice and research. *Research in Nursing and Health, 18,* 489–499.

Gross, D., & Rocissano, L. (1989). Maternal confidence in toddlerhood: Comparing preterm and fullterm groups. *Research in Nursing and Health, 12,* 1–9.

Hallas, D. (2002). Model for the successful foster care foster parent relationship. *Journal of Pediatric Health Care, 16,* 112–118.

Hallas, D., & Koslap-Petraco, M. (2004). Implementing evidence-based practice in pediatric ambulatory care centers. *Paper presented at sigma theta tau international 15th international nursing research congress and international evidence-based practice preconference, July 21, 2004.* Dublin: Ireland.

Hallas, D., & Koslap-Petraco, M. (2007). Improving psychosocial outcomes for toddlers: Teenage mothers raising toddlers: A mirrored identity crisis. *Paper presented at the sigma theta tau international honor Society of Nursing International Evidence-Based Nursing Congress, July 2007.* Vienna: Austria.

Hayes, L., Matthew, J., Copley, A., & Welsh, D. (2007). A randomized controlled trial of a mother-infant or toddler parenting program: Demonstrating effectiveness in practice. *Journal of Pediatric Psychology, 33,* 473–486 http://jpepsy.oxfordjournals.org/content/33/5/473.full.pdf+html.

Hutchings, J., Appleton, P., Smith, M., Lane, E., & Nash, S. (2002). Evaluation of two treatments for children with severe behavior problems: Child behavior and maternal mental health outcomes. *Behavioral and Cognitive Psychotherapy, 30,* 279–295.

Jemmott, L. S., Jemmott, J. B., III, Hutchinson, M. K., Cederbaum, J. A., & O'Leary, A. (2008). Sexually transmitted infection/HIV risk reduction interventions in clinical practice settings. *Journal of Obstetric, Gynecologic, & Neonatal Nursing, 37,* 137–145.

Knapp, P. E., Ammen, S., Arstein-Kerslake, C., Poulsen, M. K., & Mastergeorge, A. (2007). Feasibility of expanding services for very young children in the public mental setting. *Journal of the American Academy of Child and Adolescent Psychiatry, 46,* 152–161.

Lerner, C., & Ciervo, L. (2010). Parenting young children today: What the research tells us. Zero to Three. https://main.zerotothree.org/site/DocServer/30-4_Lerner.pdf?d.

Mendelsohn, A. L., Valdez, P. T., Flynn, V., Foley, G. M., Berkule, S. B., Tomopoulos, S., ... Dreyer, B. (2007). Use of videotaped interactions during pediatric well child care: Impact at 33 months on parenting and on child development. *Journal of Developmental Behavioral Pediatrics, 28,* 206–212 (http://www.ncbi.nlm.nih.gov/pubmed/17565287).

Surrey, J. L. (1991). The "self-in-relation": A theory of women's development. In J. V. Jordan, A. G. Kaplan, J. B. Miller, I. P. Stiver, & J. L. Surrey (Eds.), *Women's Growth in Connection: Writings from the Stone Center.* New York: The Guilford Press.

New York State Department of Health Child Health Plus web site (1985). Retrieved from http://www.health.ny.gov/health_care/child_health_plus/eligibility_and_cost.htm.

Olds, D. L., Sadler, L., & Kitzman, H. (2007). Programs for parents of infants and toddlers: Recent evidence from randomized trials. *Journal of Child Psychology and Psychiatry, 48,* 355–391.

Parents Action for Children (2006). Food and fitness matter, Raising healthy, active kids: Author. https://www.parentsaction.org.

Smith, C. L., Calkins, S. D., Keane, S. P., Anastopoulos, A. D., & Shelton, T. L. (2004). Predicting stability and change in toddler behavior problems: Contributions of maternal behavior and child gender. *Developmental Psychology, 40,* 29–42.

Sugisawa, Y., Shinohara, R., Tong, L., Tanakae, E., Watanabe, T., Onda, Y., ... Anme, T. (2010). The trajectory patterns of parenting and the social competence of toddlers: A longitudinal perspective. *Journal of Epidemiology, 20*(Suppl. 2), S459–S465 Epub 2010 Feb 23 http://www.ncbi.nlm.nih.gov/pubmed/20179370.

Walker, H. M., & Sprague, J. R. (2000). The path to school failure, delinquency, and violence: Causal factors and some potential solutions. *Interventions in School and Clinic, 35,* 67.

Watson, J. (1997). The theory of human caring: Retrospective and prospective. *Nursing Science Quarterly, 10,* 49–52.

Watson, J. (2003). Love and caring. Ethics of face and hand – An invitation to return to the heart and soul of nursing and our deep humanity. *Nursing Administration Quarterly, 27,* 197–202.

Zimmer-Gembeck, M. J., Webb, H. J., Pepping, C. A., Swan, K., Merlo, O., Skinner, E. A., ... Dunbar, M. (2015). Review: Is parent-child attachment a correlate of children's emotion regulation and coping? *International Journal of Behavioral Development,* 1–20. http://dx.doi.org/10.1177/0165025415618276.

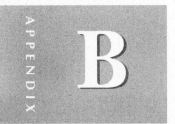

Alyssa Erikson and Betty Davies Study

Journal of Pediatric Nursing 35 (2017) 42–49

Contents lists available at ScienceDirect

Journal of Pediatric Nursing

Maintaining Integrity: How Nurses Navigate Boundaries in Pediatric Palliative Care

CrossMark

Alyssa Erikson, RN, PhD, MSN *,1, Betty Davies, RN, PhD 2

School of Nursing, Department of Family Health Care Nursing, University of California, San Francisco, San Francisco, CA, USA

ARTICLE INFO

Article history:
Received 27 August 2016
Revised 13 February 2017
Accepted 24 February 2017

Keywords:
Pediatric palliative care
Nursing
Nurses
Boundaries
Grounded theory

ABSTRACT

Purpose: To explore how nurses manage personal and professional boundaries in caring for seriously ill children and their families.

Design and methods: Using a constructivist grounded theory approach, a convenience sample of 18 registered nurses from four practice sites was interviewed using a semi-structured interview guide.

Results: Nurses across the sites engaged in a process of *maintaining integrity* whereby they integrated two competing, yet essential, aspects of their nursing role – *behaving professionally* and *connecting personally*. When skillful in both aspects, nurses were satisfied that they provided high-quality, family-centered care to children and families within a clearly defined therapeutic relationship. At times, tension existed between these two aspects and nurses attempted to *mitigate the tension*. Unsuccessful mitigation attempts led to *compromised integrity* characterized by specific behavioral and emotional indicators. Successfully mitigating the tension with strategies that prioritized their own needs and healing, nurses eventually *restored integrity*. Maintaining integrity involved a continuous effort to preserve completeness of both oneself and one's nursing practice.

Conclusions: Study findings provide a theoretical conceptualization to describe the process nurses use in navigating boundaries and contribute to an understanding for how this specialized area of care impacts health care providers.

Practice Implications: Work environments can better address the challenges of navigating boundaries through offering resources and support for nurses' emotional responses to caring for seriously ill children. Future research can further refine and expand the theoretical conceptualization of *maintaining integrity* presented in this paper and its potential applicability to other nursing specialties.

© 2017 Elsevier Inc. All rights reserved.

Pediatric palliative care (PPC) is an approach to care that emphasizes providing comprehensive care to children with life-threatening conditions and their families (American Academy of Pediatrics [AAP], 2013). In Western nations, children in need of PPC are diagnosed with life-threatening illnesses, such as congenital disorders, progressive chronic conditions, or acute, serious illnesses that may place a child at risk for premature death (Dahlin, 2013). These children are cared for in a variety of settings, most frequently in oncology and intensive care units, and in families' homes and children's hospices. Consequently, registered nurses in these settings must attend not only to children's physical and medical needs, but also to their and their families' emotional, psychosocial, and spiritual needs.

Families of seriously ill children strongly desire and deeply appreciate genuine emotional support and empathic communication from health-care providers, especially at the end of life and after their child's death (Contro, Larson, Scofield, Sourkes, & Cohen, 2002; Davies, Larson, Contro, & Cabrera, 2011; Price, Jordan, Prior, & Parkes, 2011; Stevenson, Achille, & Lugasi, 2013; Weidner et al., 2011). Moreover, families report a higher quality of care when they receive emotional support and individualized attention from health care providers caring for their child at the end of life (Heller & Solomon, 2005; Macdonald et al., 2005). Nurses caring for children at the end of life experience sadness and grief, but offering emotional support to families is an essential aspect of their practice from which they derive meaning and work satisfaction (Bloomer, O'Connor, Copnell, & Endacott, 2015; Cook et al., 2012; Kain, 2013; Reid, 2013; Stayer, 2016). It is to be expected that nurses who practice in these emotionally charged situations confront issues related to

* Corresponding author: Alyssa Erikson, RN, PhD, MSN.
E-mail address: aerikson@csumb.edu (A. Erikson).
1 Present address: California State University, Monterey Bay, Seaside, CA, 93955.
2 Present address: School of Nursing, University of Victoria, Victoria, British Columbia, Canada.

http://dx.doi.org/10.1016/j.pedn.2017.02.031
0882-5963/© 2017 Elsevier Inc. All rights reserved.

A. Erikson, B. Davies / Journal of Pediatric Nursing 35 (2017) 42–49   43

professional boundaries but little is known about how nurses manage professional and personal boundaries within the context of PPC. The purpose of this paper is to describe how pediatric nurses defined boundaries and present a theoretical conceptualization of an identified process for managing boundaries, entitled maintaining integrity.

Background

Nurses offer emotional support to patients and families by establishing a therapeutic relationship, defined as "one that allows nurses to apply their professional knowledge, skills, abilities, and experiences towards meeting the health needs of the patient" (The National Council of State Boards of Nursing [NCSBN], 2014, p. 3). The therapeutic relationship occurs along a continuum of professional boundaries which are "the spaces between the nurse's power and the patient's vulnerability and which exists between the extreme ends of under and over-involvement (NCSBN, 2014, p. 3). The NCSBN advises nurses that boundary violations primarily occur in the over-involved end on the continuum when the nurse's needs supersede the patient's or the family's needs, such as when discussing intimate or personal issues with a patient, spending more time than necessary with a particular patient, or showing favoritism. Aligned with the NCSBN's guidelines, some authors caution nurses not to get too close, emotionally attached, or over-involved with patients and their families (Anewalt, 2009; Pate & Barshay, 2012; Roberts, Fenton, & Barnard, 2015). However, none of these guidelines describe how nurses themselves perceive and manage boundaries. That is, what do "spaces between the nurse's power and the patient's vulnerability" look like in actual day-to-day practice?

Pediatric nurses, in a phenomenological study exploring therapeutic boundaries (Totka, 1996), experienced an intrapersonal struggle in finding an appropriate level of involvement with families. The research team wrestled with identifying the point when instances of over-involvement became "crossing the line" because sometimes families and nurses mutually benefitted from over-involvement. Similarly, other researchers (Cook et al., 2012; Reid, 2013) reported that nurses caring for dying children defined boundaries by their level of involvement with families and acknowledged that over-involvement periodically occurred; they too were challenged in maintaining the fine line between involvement and detachment. These studies suggest that professional boundaries are more complex and layered with nuances than current NCSBN (2014) guidelines indicate.

Other reports of nurses caring for seriously ill or dying children contributed to an understanding of the emotional, more personal, aspects of nurses' work. Working with seriously ill or dying children triggered nurses' reflections about their personal assumptions and beliefs about self, life, death, past unresolved losses, future anticipated losses of loved ones, and loss of self through death (Papadatou & Bellali, 2002; Yam, Rossiter, & Cheung, 2001). Nurses responded to patients' deaths with grief, sadness, hurting, moral distress, struggling and suffering. These elicited emotions can lead to compassion fatigue, which is state of feeling physically, emotionally, and mentally exhausted to provide adequate nursing care (Berger, Polivka, Smoot, & Owens, 2015). Burnout is a component of compassion fatigue and associated with nurses' grief experience and work satisfaction (Adwan, 2014; Meyer, Li, Klaristenfeld, & Gold, 2015). Burnout can also result from moral distress (Rushton, Kaszniak, & Halifax, 2013), which is provoked by emotionally-wrought situations, such as aggressive treatments that are against the patient's best interest or flawed interdisciplinary communication (Trotochaud, Coleman, Krawiecki, & McCracken, 2015). Moreover, emotional responses can persist, such as memories of patients' deaths continuing to "haunt" nurses years after the experience (Papadatou & Bellali, 2002; Rashotte, Fothergill-Bourbonnais, & Chamberlain, 1997). Olson et al. (1998) reported that pediatric oncology nurses openly wept when recounting their lowest point, or nadir experience, even when these instances happened many years earlier. Caring for seriously ill children who may die affects pediatric nurses on a personal level.

Understanding how nurses manage professional boundaries must also include examining their personal boundaries, thus the overall aim of our study was to explore how nurses perceived and managed professional and personal boundaries. In this paper, we describe how pediatric nurses defined boundaries and present a theoretical conceptualization of how the nurses engaged in a process of maintaining integrity to manage boundaries.

Design and Methods

Because little was known about how pediatric nurses manage professional and personal boundaries, we selected a qualitative research design, specifically grounded theory (GT). GT focuses on processes and enables development of a theory or theoretical conceptualization grounded in participants' own words, experiences, and descriptions (Charmaz, 2014). Approval to conduct the study was obtained from the institutional review boards at the major university with which the researchers were affiliated and at each study site.

Recruitment

To enhance sampling variation, the principal investigator (PI) recruited registered nurses (RNs) from two sites: a freestanding pediatric palliative care center and an academic tertiary-care children's hospital, both situated in a large, metropolitan area in the Western United States. The nine-bed center is independent from a hospital and offers respite, transitional, and end-of-life care to children with life-threatening conditions. In the children's hospital, nurses were recruited from the three units where the most deaths occur (Institute of Medicine [IOM], 2003): the oncology unit, intensive care nursery (ICN), and pediatric intensive care unit (PICU).

Using purposeful sampling, RNs were recruited through approved flyers posted in each setting and through snowball sampling. The inclusion criterion was that participants were employed as RNs in one of the four study settings. Interested RNs emailed or phoned the PI to schedule a mutually convenient time and place to meet for an interview, most often in a private area at their workplace before or after their shift. Consent, along with demographic data, was obtained at this time. Following the Consolidated Criteria for Reporting Qualitative Studies (COREQ), the female PI, interviewed all participants following training in qualitative methodologies, specifically grounded theory (Tong, Sainsbury, & Craig, 2007). The PI is an RN and established a relationship with the four study sites prior to participant enrollment through introducing the study and its purpose at staff meetings. The PI had previously worked as an RN on one of the sites prior to the study, which prompted an interest in this study area.

Data Collection

The sample included 18 RNs (10 from the PPC center, 3 from the oncology unit, 3 from the ICN, and 2 from the PICU). The participants were predominantly female (89%), White (83%), with an overall average age of 39 years. Nearly all (84%) had a BS or MS, had worked in their respective settings for an average of nearly 4 years, and their years of nursing experience ranged from 2.5 to 44 years with a mean of nearly 16 years (see Table 1). Although two males (11%) completed interviews, we refer to all participants by the female gender to maintain participant anonymity. The PI conducted interviews using a semi-structured guide with open-ended questions. To set a comfortable tone, all interviews started with a neutral prompt: "Tell me about how you came to work here." Other sample questions included: "When you tell others of your job, what do you tell them?", "Describe a family or child you cared for that stands out in your memory and tell me the story of caring for them," and "Describe how you cope with the emotionally stressful part of your job." Interviews ranged from 45 to 75 min, were audiotaped, and transcribed verbatim by a professional transcription

Table 1
Sample characteristics.

Demographic Data (N = 18)	n (%) or M (range)
Work Setting	
End of life facility	10 (56%)
Children's hospital	8 (44%)
Hem/onc/bmt unit	3 (17%)
PICU	2 (11%)
ICN	3 (17%)
Gender	
Female	16 (89%)
Male	2 (11%)
Ethnicity	
White	15 (83%)
Black	1 (5%)
Other	2 (11%)
Age in years (n = 15)[a]	
Overall	39.2 (25–59)
End of life facility	44.0 (29–59)
Children's hospital	27.4 (25–42)
Education	
Diploma	1 (5%)
Associate's	2 (11%)
Bachelor's	10 (56%)
Master's	5 (28%)
Years in work setting	
Overall	3.79 (0.4–15.5)
End of life facility	1.77 (0.4–2.75)
Children's hospital	6.31 (2.5–17.0)
Years of nursing experience	
Overall	15.69 (2.5–44.0)
End of life facility	21.40 (6.0–44.0)
Children's hospital	8.56 (2.5–29.0)
Years of pediatric experience	
Overall	12.75 (2.5–42.0)
End of life facility	16.10 (3.0–42.0)
Children's hospital	8.56 (2.5–29.0)

[a] Three participants declined to state age.

service. All identifying personal and patient information were removed from the transcriptions. The PI cross-checked and confirmed transcripts with the original recordings for accuracy and then destroyed original recordings.

Data Analysis

In accordance with constructivist GT principles (Charmaz, 2014), we began data analysis with the first interview and continued throughout data collection. Line-by-line or chunk-by-chunk analysis resulted in initial codes that identified actions in the data, such as "managing pain,", "feeling attachment," and "taking a break." Salient and significant initial codes were then clustered into focused codes such as "suppressing undesired emotion,", "feeling tension" or "connecting to patients and families." These codes were later clustered into groups in the process of axial coding, which link codes together for further exploration and analysis. Examples of axial codes are "displaying emotion", "maintaining professionalism," and "supporting families." Constant comparison of the codes, categories, themes, and narratives highlighted similarities and differences between and among participants' stories and facilitated the examination of relationships within the data. As analysis progressed, a conceptualization evolved and was further refined through ongoing data collection and analysis.

Trustworthiness

We adhered to established strategies used in qualitative research to address trustworthiness (Polit & Beck, 2016); prolonged engagement, peer review, and member checking. The researchers addressed reflexivity through writing and analyzing memos throughout the research process which explored emerging themes with researchers' values and beliefs. The PI presented findings to three participants who affirmed

that the conceptualization reflected their experience. We followed GT principles to ensure the resulting theoretical conceptualization was grounded in nurses' words and experiences. Data saturation was achieved when new interviews added no new information.

Results

From our analysis, we identified that the pediatric nurses across the four study settings engaged in a process of *maintaining integrity* as they navigated personal and professional boundaries. "Integrity" referred to nurses' sense of wholeness and of being true to oneself that they felt when they successfully navigated their professional and personal boundaries. We describe how nurses characterized personal and professional boundaries and then present the theoretical conceptualization of the process of *maintaining integrity*.

Personal and Professional Boundaries

In describing their work with seriously ill or dying children, all nurses spontaneously mentioned words associated with boundaries, such as "limits," "crossing lines," or what they deemed "appropriate/inappropriate behavior." Most participants defined, constructed, and regulated their own boundaries, indicating that the process was highly individualized. Some nurses remembered being warned about boundaries in nursing school, but at the beginning of their careers, most participants felt overwhelmed and confused about how to set boundaries: "As a new nurse it was very, very hard distinguishing boundaries." Nurses calibrated their boundaries according to each particular child or parent:

You kind of have to feel out each family. We have so many cultures that come through, that each family lets you know how comfortable they are with touch and medical staff. You have to feel each situation out and see what's appropriate for that family. Even though maybe I'm more touchy, I have to recognize maybe this person isn't as touchy and it's okay to have more boundaries and let them have their personal space.

With experience over time, especially with patients' deaths, nurses became more skilled in defining and negotiating boundaries. Particular incidents stood out and participants clearly remembered caring for the first child that died: "I remember the very first patient I ever had die. The exact date, the time, just everything about it." For some nurses, these first experiences were especially memorable because they had become too close or attached to the child and/or parents and were distressed when the child died. Feeling involved with patients or families on a more personal and emotional level prompted nurses to re-negotiate personal boundaries about how personally invested they became to future patients. It was a balance for some nurses to determine how close they became to patients while still protecting their self:

I think it's taken me this long to really figure out how I can protect myself and be empathetic, but not suffer because of it. Because there was a period of time where I didn't really know that fine dance of how to do that well.

When speaking about personal boundaries, nurses focused on behaviors that buffered them from the emotional effects of their work. These behaviors included keeping a distance from patients and families and strictly maintaining a separation between their personal life and work. Nurses defined personal boundaries by how much they opened up when disclosing personal information with children or parents and by limiting the amount of information they shared about themselves, thus keeping their focus of the care of the patients and parents, "No matter how close to them [the families] I am, it was always mainly about them."

In describing professional boundaries, nurses usually referred to professional codes of conduct, such as patient safety principles, treating patients and families fairly, and ethical behavior. They used the

A. Erikson, B. Davies / Journal of Pediatric Nursing 35 (2017) 42–49   45

qualifying words "appropriate" or "inappropriate" in describing professional boundaries, most commonly in reference to getting close to patients or parents: "You always are afraid when you say you get close to a patient that you're going beyond the appropriate boundaries." Nurses could not specifically identify the source for what or who dictated appropriate actions, but mentioned that nursing school, professional discourse, administrative guidelines, personal opinions, or articles in the literature potentially influenced them. Across sites, nurses were not aware of any clear administrative rules about professional behavior, such as bringing special gifts to patients, seeing patients outside of work, or assisting a family in finding housing. Nurses discovered a rule existed, however, when they were reprimanded for crossing a line.

Maintaining Integrity

From our analysis, we identified the process of *maintaining integrity* whereby nurses integrated two competing, yet essential, aspects of their nursing role – *behaving professionally* and *connecting personally* (See Fig. 1). When skillful in both aspects, nurses were satisfied that they were providing high-quality, family-centered care to children and families within a clearly defined therapeutic relationship. At times, tension existed between these two aspects and nurses attempted to *mitigate the tension*. Unsuccessful mitigation attempts led to *compromised integrity* characterized by specific behavioral and emotional indicators. Successfully mitigating the tension with strategies that

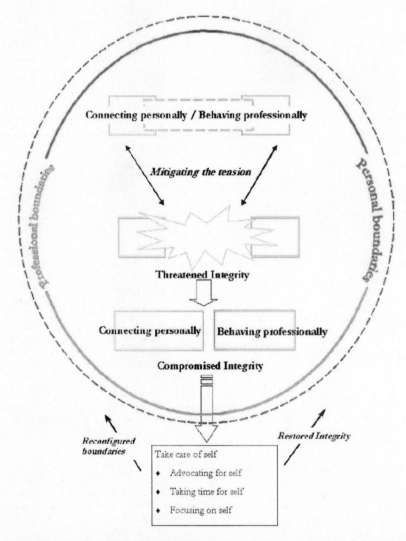

Fig. 1. A theoretical conceptualization of the process of maintaining integrity. We identified the process of *maintaining integrity* whereby nurses integrated two competing, yet essential, aspects of their nursing role – *behaving professionally* and *connecting personally*. These two aspects reside within personal and professional boundaries, indicated by the red and blue circular lines. Analysis revealed that personal and professional boundaries are not separate and often blur together, which is represented by the purple dotted line as the outer edge of the circle. Inside the circle, *connecting personally* (yellow box) and *behaving professionally* (blue box) coexist together (dotted green line) and when skillful in both aspects, nurses were satisfied that they were providing high-quality, family-centered care. At times, tension existed between these two aspects and nurses attempted to *mitigate the tension*, but if they were unable to mitigate the tension, this led to *threatened integrity*. Unresolved *threatened integrity* could lead to *compromised integrity*, represented in the figure as the *connecting personally* and *behaving professionally* boxes independent from one another and no longer coexisting. Nurses could no longer skillfully integrate both aspects in their practice. Through focusing on strategies of self-care, nurses could eventually *restored integrity* with reconfigured boundaries and entered back into the process.

46   *A. Erikson, B. Davies / Journal of Pediatric Nursing 35 (2017) 42–49*

prioritized their own needs and healing, nurses eventually *restored integrity* with reconfigured boundaries. Maintaining integrity involved a continuous effort to preserve completeness of both oneself and one's nursing practice.

Behaving Professionally

As noted earlier, we identified professional boundaries in nurses' interviews when they deemed actions as appropriate or inappropriate. Nurses most commonly described behaving professionally as keeping an emotional separation from patients and families. They kept this distance to abide by professional codes of conduct (e.g. not favoring particular patients or families), focus their care on patients' and families' needs, or protect themselves from distressing emotional responses to a child's death. Nurses labeled inappropriate professional behaviors as "crossing the line," such as visiting patients during their off time, socializing with families outside of work, assisting families with personal favors, or buying presents for patients. One nurse described feeling tempted to integrate patients into her own family: "I wish I could take one of the kids with me over to my family's house and hang out with my nieces and nephews like they're a part of my family. That would be crossing boundaries to me." Nurses also perceived excessive displays of emotion in front of families as inappropriate professional behavior.

Connecting Personally

Connecting personally occurred through nurses engaging with patients and families, providing emotional support, empathizing, and in some cases, forming attachments to particular families. Connections deepened during patients' recurrent and long hospitalizations, which allowed for space and time to forge relationships. Over these protracted admissions, nurses got to know children and parents on a more personal level: "I knew everything about that kid, just everything about him. His parents' names, how long they were married. I know all about them." Commonalities between nurses and particular children or parents, such as similar backgrounds, life experiences, or ages of their child, intensified connections: "It's true what they say. If an [ill child] is the same age as your kid's age, you think it could be your kid." Forming attachments occurred when nurses became personally invested in a child's or family's welfare, such as when they could not stop thinking about patients outside of work, volunteered to stay after their shifts to continue caring for a family, visited patients on their days off, or brought special gifts to children and families. In reflecting on these experiences, nurses often were aware that they violated boundaries but could not help but become attached to families.

Threatened Integrity

Behaving professionally and connecting personally had competing goals; where one seeks separation, the other strives for engagement, thus creating a natural tension. Usually, this tension did not disrupt nurses' day-to-day work but other times, nurses acutely experienced the tension and felt it threatened their integrity. These times of tension centered on 1) separating work from personal time; 2) being a friend vis a vis a caregiver; 3) crying in front of families; and 4) experiencing ethical or moral distress.

Nurses varied in how they perceived the separation between work and personal time. Some nurses held a clearly delineated line, whereas others perceived a natural overlap between work and personal time. Tension typically arose when parents invited nurses to attend a special event for their child. These invitations tested professional boundaries because nurses wanted to support families (i.e. connect personally) but attending these events would be on their personal time and outside of their nursing role. Some nurses mitigated this tension by vigilantly segregating their work and personal lives, partly as a self-protection

strategy from overwhelming emotions and to sustain a clear professional boundary:

> For me, it needs to be separate. I couldn't do what I do if it was personal for me. Like I took her [patient's] death hard, but I don't think ever as hard as I know other people have taken deaths and it's because I never let them in fully. Because I know that, if I did, I wouldn't be able to do it.

In contrast, other nurses had difficulty compartmentalizing their work and personal lives. Instead, they perceived such things as sending a card to a family to acknowledge their child's birthday or day of death as a continuation of their professional role and not as a boundary violation. Yet, when they were invited to a child's special event - all of which occurred during their personal time - they still struggled with the decision to accept the invitation or not.

Tension also arose from when nurses were deciding to attend a child's funeral or memorial. Nurses who strictly separated their work from their personal time did not attend: "If you go to the funeral, then you're mixing your personal life, and your work life. The family is seeing me outside of work, but I'm still the nurse." Other nurses perceived their attendance as continued support for the family. In the ICN, for example, nurses perceived that knowing the baby from birth through death was a reason to attend the funeral: "We're there at the beginning and we're there at the end." However, across settings, when nurses experienced multiple deaths in a short amount of time, the tension about attending funerals increased. Attending multiple funerals was emotionally draining and sometimes personally disturbing. At the PPC center, families can hold memorial services there and this made it possible for these nurses to attend services as part of their job, thereby lessening the tension between their professional and personal lives.

Tension between connecting personally and behaving professionally also influenced how nurses defined their role in relationships with families as a friend or a caregiver. Connecting personally created the potential for nurses to befriend patients or their parents, ultimately compromising their therapeutic relationship. Most nurses mitigated this tension by consciously focusing on their caregiving role:

> Your role [in the hospital] is as a caregiver, that's your job. It's not a mutual relationship. And, to enter into that relationship outside work – are you expected to continue the caregiving role or is it going to become a mutual friendship?

Other nurses, however, classified some activities as part of their caregiving role. These gestures, such as checking in with parents on their day off, sending cards to families after a child's death, or helping a parent find housing, supported and met the needs of patients and their parents.

Crying in front of families also caused tension for participants. An inherent expectation of behaving professionally was to refrain from crying, yet connecting personally expectedly triggered nurses' emotions. Nurses, across settings, acknowledged that crying was a natural response to the gravity of their work: "There's nothing normal about a two month old dying." Nurses mitigated this tension by concluding that crying was a normal, human response to the loss of a child's life and bearing witness to the family's grief: "If you're distraught, you're distraught. And that's okay because you're human and you're supposed to be emotional." In general, nurses perceived that crying was acceptable but uncontrollable bawling was inappropriate and unprofessional because this excessive display of emotion shifted the focus from the family onto the nurse. A few participants regretfully remembered a time early in their career where the family had to comfort *them*. Nurses continually navigated a fine line between appropriate and inappropriate crying in front of families.

Finally, situations of moral distress increased the tension between professional and personal aspects, particularly for nurses working in the hospital settings when they administered aggressive treatments to children at the end-of-life and which they perceived as futile. Across

A. Erikson, B. Davies / Journal of Pediatric Nursing 35 (2017) 42–49 47

settings, however, nurses experienced moral distress when they felt personally conflicted about a plan of care, especially when a procedure was not aligned with patients' wishes or when they implemented or witnessed procedures that caused pain or prolonged suffering. They mitigated their own distress by reframing procedures as part of their professional responsibilities:

> I think the areas where I struggle the most with are when they do want to be really, really aggressive and drag the child through transfusions and IV chemo and keep on going and going and going. And you see this decline and the suffering of a child. But I just have to still be professional.

Many nurses noted that these experiences distressed them for many years afterward.

Compromised Integrity

For the most part, nurses successfully mitigated the tension between behaving professionally and connecting personally. However, when they were not able to mitigate the tension, it compromised their integrity, or feeling of wholeness, identified in our analysis by words such as "immobilized," "heavy," "burned out," as if they were "hitting a wall," or "weighed down". Physically, nurses described feeling fatigue, headaches or general malaise and emotionally they described grief, anger, or hopelessness. Periods of compromised integrity negatively affected both their work and their personal lives. Children's deaths, especially when multiple patients died in a short period of time, often compounded their sense of compromised integrity: "You get that lethargy of grief. It affects your heart and soul, so you just feel weighed down." They coped by distancing themselves: "After you get really connected to a few [children] and then you lose them, I think you kind of put up a wall…you invest so much that it's emotionally draining." One nurse described a time of being burned out and thus distancing from her patients: "It was almost like you were there, you did your job, and you left. There was nothing else." Nurses were distressed by distancing because they were not providing professional, compassionate care. Outside of work, nurses dreamt of dead patients, cried uncontrollably, or withdrew from family or friends. They did not want to work and interact with patients, parents or colleagues: "I really enjoy my job…I get a lot of fulfillment from it and I got to the point where I didn't want to come to work. Every day was a struggle." Moreover, nurses felt they must push through these periods of compromised integrity and continue to work despite their pain, which only deepened their distress. In reflecting on these experiences, nurses labeled their physical and emotional indicators as "red flags," and that they served as a warning to take a break.

Integrity Restored

To restore integrity, nurses realized that they needed to step back and take care of themselves:

> I was like, 'Oh gosh, I'm exhausted and drained'. And, I remember I went to sleep and I was dreaming of the baby, and all these things that stick with you because you didn't deal with it yourself. You were trying to help everyone else deal with it that you're like, 'Oh wow, I need to do some self-care'.

Nurses engaged in self-care by taking time for, advocating for, and focusing on themselves. They took time off which ranged from taking a short break during a shift to a month-long leave for vacation, teaching, or volunteer work. In advocating for themselves, nurses recognized their own needs and limits and requested to be reassigned from an emotionally draining case or sought help from colleagues. Nurses focused on themselves by engaging in gratifying experiences outside of the work setting, such as attending church, scheduling massages or facials, taking quiet walks, exercising, seeing a therapist, spending time

with family and friends, and attending social events with their colleagues.

Employing these strategies restored nurses' integrity or sense of wholeness so they returned to work feeling capable of providing quality care once again. Restoring integrity often meant reconfiguring personal or professional boundaries. For example, if nurses felt that they had been too close to patients or families, they adjusted boundaries so they could engage with patients and provide necessary emotional support, but be less personally involved. Despite years of nursing experience in palliative care, even veteran nurses still experienced periods of compromised integrity that required ongoing refinement of their personal and professional boundaries: "I am growing and learning how to that better every day". When compromised integrity was restored, nurses felt satisfied and rewarded in their work. They enjoyed the challenges of working with serious ill children and families, rather than feeling overburdened and overwhelmed. They acknowledged the emotional personal stress of caring for children who died, and simultaneously valued their professional work as fulfilling:

> This can be a very difficult place to be, but it still can be a phenomenal place of joy and appreciation of the moment. It has been a true life lesson for me – just to stop and smell the roses. Sometimes, literally. Stopping with a child and picking flowers. And maybe in three days, they're gone. And the flowers are gone too.

Discussion

The intent of this inquiry was to explore how pediatric nurses manage boundaries when caring for seriously ill or dying children. The analysis of the data enabled us to develop a conceptualization indicating that nurses simultaneously engaged in connecting personally and behaving professionally which could create tension and at times, compromised integrity. Nurses considered boundaries at all stages of their career and particular patient experiences affected how they created and maintained boundaries. All nurses agreed on blatant boundary violations in nursing practice, like emotional, physical or sexual abuse. Study findings reflected nuances and intricacies of balancing professional and personal boundaries, which was a highly individualized, intrapersonal process for nurses and a more complex process than simply following a set of rules.

Our data sheds new light on two aspects of maintaining boundaries: 1) Managing boundaries is more complex than guidelines or rules that imply a predictable and straight-forward patient situation, and 2) maintaining integrity for pediatric nurses must take into account the unique nature of the nurses' therapeutic relationship with parents and children.

This study is one of the first to include nurses across multiple settings and with nurses from a PPC center and provides insight into how nurses construct, perceive, and then negotiate professional boundaries in caring for seriously ill children. Findings revealed that nurses continually adapted to new and challenging situations that redefined their boundaries. The NCSBN (2014) and other authors provide a standard on professional boundaries for nurses to follow, but do not address *how* nurses can do so or recognize the complex nature of boundaries (Holder & Schenthal, 2007; Mendes, 2014; Thompson, 2007; Wright, 2006). These publications connote a fixed, singular, and rigid boundary that assumes predictable patient situations; whereas, our findings offer a different perspective that takes into account the personal aspect of nursing practice. When caring for children and families, the nurse connected personally in conjunction with behaving professionally.

Connecting personally and behaving professionally created a natural tension, which was evident when nurses discriminated between caregiving and friendship behaviors. Some nurses perceived contact with parents outside of the work setting as a violation of professional boundaries, yet, other nurses stated that staying in contact with parents whose child died and/or attending a funeral are valuable sources of support for grieving parents, which is supported by prior research (Macdonald et

48 *A. Erikson, B. Davies / Journal of Pediatric Nursing 35 (2017) 42–49*

al., 2005; Stevenson et al., 2013). These findings are in contrast to the NCSBN guidelines and the American Nursing Association (ANA)'s Code of Ethics (2015) which counsel nurses about forming inappropriate relationships, such as friendships, with patients or family members. The issue may be in how guidelines and nurses define friendships and what attributes characterize friendships. The prevalence of social media (e.g. Facebook or Instagram) further complicates the issue because nurses and family members have another medium to share aspects of their personal lives. The Code of Ethics specifically addresses receiving gifts as a boundary violation. Notably, nurses in our study described giving gifts, attending funerals, crying in front of families, providing futile treatments, and friendships as sources of tension relating to boundaries, but did not mention receiving gifts.

The NCSBN guideline on professional boundaries discusses under-involvement, which was evident in our findings when nurses distanced themselves in response to feeling overwhelmed with emotional demands of their work. This phenomenon has been described in previous studies for how nurses cope after the death of pediatric patients, especially in feeling that they cannot give of themselves and respond by disconnecting from families (Davies et al., 1996; Papadatou, Martinson, & Chung, 2001; Rashotte et al., 1997; Reid, 2013). NCSBN characterizes under-involvement as a professional boundary violation, but our findings suggest that it should be regarded as an indicator that nurses are experiencing distress or difficulty in their work. As a signal for compromised integrity, distancing is in line with a growing literature on compassion fatigue, moral distress and burnout in pediatric nurses (Adwan, 2014; Berger et al., 2015; Trotochaud et al., 2015; Zander, Hutton, & King, 2010). The danger is that distancing might progress to feelings of depersonalization (Gallagher & Gormley, 2009; Yam et al., 2001), which is detrimental to not only patient care but to nurses' personal lives. When their integrity was compromised, most of the participants in our study ignored the indicators and pressed on, compounding their distress. Eventually, often with the help of a supportive work environment and self-reflection, many realized a change was necessary and they intentionally engaged in self-care. The result was reintegration, accompanied by new knowledge in how to better negotiate their professional and personal boundaries. Guidelines often characterize boundaries as a simplified list of inappropriate behavior and would be more helpful to nurses if they included a more complete discussion of the nuanced process of navigating boundaries.

Our findings showed that the nurses came to realize that every patient and family situation is unique because of the element of *human* interaction and boundaries must be open to modification to adapt to each situation. We do not argue that nurses should not have boundaries, but rather for consideration of the human relationship that is at the center of nursing practice, and is a goal for PPC (IOM, 2003). Clearly, certain unprofessional behaviors threaten or violate patients' needs, such as neglect, abuse, or disclosing highly personal information. Participants, however, did not talk about "crossing the line" in these extreme ways. Rather, they navigated boundaries in terms of their relationship to patients and families in ongoing human interaction, and in line with Milton's (2008) view that "boundaries exist in the labeling of the professional role of the nurse as something between professionalism and friendship" (p. 29). Professional boundaries were primarily the limits they placed on maintaining a professional and care-giving relationship, where their focus centered on attending to patient and family needs.

Limitations

The majority of participants in the study were female, white and had a considerable number of years of nursing experience. The first author previously worked as an RN at one of the study sites and worked with some of the study participants. This may have influenced how these participants answered interview questions. The authors, however, were aware of this potential bias during the course of analysis and noted no major differences between their experiences and the others.

Additionally, over half the sample was recruited from the PPC center, more than the nurses from the hospital units combined, despite a significantly smaller population of nurses working in the PPC center. These nurses were more willing to participate and easier to recruit. Since the study was advertised as a PPC study, participants may have perceived PPC as integral to their care and may have been more comfortable discussing death and dying compared to non-volunteers. This would apply especially to the nurses working in the PPC center as dying and death are frequent and open topics of discussion. However, this study is one of the first to include nurses across multiple settings, including both acute care and a PPC center. Thus, findings provide insights about the similarity of nurses' experiences in how they construct, perceive, and then negotiate professional boundaries in caring for seriously ill children. Despite this limitation, the findings present implications for practice and research.

Practice Implications

Findings suggest that when caring for children who are seriously ill, nurses' continually engage in an internally regulated process of navigating professional and personal boundaries that are flexible and adaptable. Thus, findings have implications for both undergraduate and continuing education programs where educators should create opportunities for students to learn about the process of maintaining integrity. Preparing nurses to provide palliative care should include how to manage attachments to patients and families, deal with work-related emotions, cope with moral or ethical distress, recognize common emotional or behavioral indicators which signal compromised integrity, and how to implement strategies for restoring integrity, while accounting for the human relationships that develop among patients, families, and providers. Established palliative care training programs can serve as models since they include curriculum about providers' emotional responses and self-care (Education in Palliative and End-of-Life Care [EPEC], n.d; End of Life Nursing Education Consortium [ELNEC], 2016; The Initiative for Pediatric Palliative Care [IPPC], 2014).

Additionally, newer nurses may feel more supported within work settings if they understand that working in palliative care can elicit a range of emotions and are taught strategies and resources for coping with these emotions. Findings also point to implications for developing a milieu in the workplace where discussions can occur comfortably and that acknowledges the challenges of caring for seriously ill children who may die. For example, staffing levels should support nurses caring for dying patients and enable them to have a break between a patient's death and a new admission. Nurses could be reimbursed for attending memorial or funeral services to more clearly frame this act as part of their caregiving role and reduce professional/personal boundary tension arising from the dilemma of attending funerals on their personal time. The value of peer support is clear (Cook et al., 2012; Forster & Haiz, 2015; Reid, 2013) and models of support are available (Ewing & Carter, 2004; Macpherson, 2008; Rushton et al., 2006).

Because this is one of the first studies to describe how nurses navigate boundaries in pediatric palliative care, more research is needed to better understand the process and explore beneficial interventions to support nurses. PPC research has grown substantially in the last two decades, but the impact on health care providers in this field is not fully understood. Further studies could address this impact and identify barriers or facilitators for providing optimal care. Insights could also be drawn from a study including both nurses and parents to understand how each side perceives boundaries. Study participants did not explicitly address social media, which is a rapidly advancing and pervasive topic that is under-studied in the nursing literature. It warrants further research aimed at exploring personal and professional boundaries and the ethical nature of nurses connecting on social media platforms with patients and their families. Finally, this study recruited nurses from multiple settings, but it may be helpful in future research to recruit nurses

A. Erikson, B. Davies / Journal of Pediatric Nursing 35 (2017) 42–49

from additional settings where children are seriously ill, such as in cardiology, another type of hospice or a home-care/hospice agency.

In conclusion, the aim of this study was to understand how nurses managed personal and professional boundaries, which is an understudied area in pediatric palliative care. Study findings provide a theoretical conceptualization to describe a process nurses used in navigating boundaries and contribute to an understanding for how this specialized area of care impacts health care providers. Nurses working in PPC settings, both in and out of the hospital, can benefit from early recognition of the behavioral and emotional indicators of compromised integrity. Work environments can better address the challenges of navigating boundaries through offering resources and support for nurses' emotional responses to caring for seriously ill children. Future research can further refine and expand the theoretical conceptualization of *maintaining integrity* and its potential applicability to other nursing specialties.

Acknowledgment

This work was supported by the Betty Irene Moore Pre-doctoral Fellowship at the University of California, San Francisco.

References

Adwan, J. Z. (2014). Pediatric nurses' grief experience, burnout and job satisfaction. *Journal of Pediatric Nursing, 29*(4), 329–336. http://dx.doi.org/10.1016/j.pedn.2014.01.011 328p.

American Academy of Pediatrics Section on Hospice and Palliative Medicine and Committee on Hospital Care (2013). Pediatric palliative care and hospice care commitments, guidelines and recommendations. *Pediatrics, 132*(5), 966–972. http://dx.doi.org/10.1542/peds.2013-2731.

American Nurses Association (2015). *Code of ethics for nurses with interpretive statements.* Silver Springs, MD: American Nurses Association.

Anewalt, P. (2009). Fired up or burned out? Understanding the importance of professional boundaries in home healthcare and hospice. *Home Healthcare Nurse, 27*(10), 590–597. http://dx.doi.org/10.1097/01.NHH.0000364181.02400.8c.

Berger, J., Polivka, B., Smoot, E. A., & Owens, H. (2015). Compassion fatigue in pediatric nurses. *Journal of Pediatric Nursing, 30*(6), e11–e17. http://dx.doi.org/10.1016/j.pedn.2015.02.005. 11p.

Bloomer, M. J., O'Connor, M., Copnell, B., & Endacott, R. (2015). Nursing care for the families of the dying child/infant in paediatric and neonatal ICU: Nurses' emotional talk and sources of discomfort. A mixed methods study. *Australian critical care: official journal of the Confederation of Australian Critical Care Nurses, 28*(2), 87–92. http://dx.doi.org/10.1016/j.aucc.2015.01.002

Charmaz, K. (2014). Constructing Grounded Theory. London: SAGE Publications Ltd.

Contro, N., Larson, J., Scofield, S., Sourkes, B., & Cohen, H. (2002). Family perspectives on the quality of pediatric palliative care. *Archives of Pediatrics & Adolescent Medicine, 156*(1), 14–19.

Cook, K. A., Mott, S., Lawrence, P., Jablonski, J., Grady, M. R., Norton, D., ... Connor, J. A. (2012). Coping while caring for the dying child: Nurses' experiences in an acute care setting. *Journal of Pediatric Nursing, 27*(4), e11–e21. http://dx.doi.org/10.1016/j.pedn.2011.05.010.

Dahlin, C. (2013). Clinical practice guidelines for quality palliative care. Retrieved from Pittsburg, Pennsylvania. http://www.nationalconsensusproject.org/NCP_Clinical_Practice_Guidelines_3rd_Edition.pdf.

Davies, B., Cook, K., O'Loane, M., Clarke, D., MacKenzie, B., Stutzer, C., ... McCormick, J. (1996). Caring for dying children: Nurses' experience. *Pediatric Nursing, 22*(6), 500–507 (508p).

Davies, B., Larson, J., Contro, N., & Cabrera, A. P. (2011). Perceptions of discrimination among Mexican American families of seriously ill children. *Journal of Palliative Medicine, 14*(1), 71–76. http://dx.doi.org/10.1089/jpm.2010.0315

End-of-Life Nursing Education Consortium (2016). ELNEC Fact Sheet. Retrieved from http://www.aacn.nche.edu/elnec/about/fact-sheet.

EPEC: Education in Palliative and End-of-Life Care. (n.d.). Curricula: Pediatrics. Retreived from http://bioethics.northwestern.edu/programs/epec/curricula/pediatrics.html.

Ewing, A., & Carter, B. S. (2004). Pediatric ethics, issues, & commentary. Once again, Vanderbilt NICU in Nashville leads the way in nurses' emotional support. *Pediatric Nursing, 30*(6), 471–472 (472p).

Forster, E., & Haiz, A. (2015). Paediatric death and dying: exploring coping strategies of health professionals and perceptions of support provision. *International Journal of Palliative Nursing, 21*(6), 294–301 (298p).

Gallagher, R., & Gormley, D. K. (2009). Perceptions of stress, burnout, and support systems in pediatric bone marrow transplantation nursing. *Clinical Journal of Oncology Nursing, 13*(6), 681–685. http://dx.doi.org/10.1188/09.CJON.681-685.

Heller, K. S., & Solomon, M. Z. (2005). Continuity of care and caring: what matters to parents of children with life-threatening conditions. *Journal of Pediatric Nursing, 20*(5), 335–346.

Holder, K. V., & Schenthal, S. J. (2007). Watch your step: nursing and professional boundaries. *Nursing Management, 38*(2), 24–29.

Institute of Medicine. Committee on Palliative and End-of-Life Care for Children and Their Families (2003L). In M. J. Field, & R. E. Behrman (Eds.), *When children die: improving palliative and end-of-life care for children and their families.* Washington, D.C.: National Academies Press.

Kain, V. J. (2013). An exploration of the grief experiences of neonatal nurses: a focus group study. *Journal of Neonatal Nursing, 19*(2), 80–88.

Macdonald, M. E., Liben, S., Carnevale, F. A., Rennick, J. E., Wolf, S. L., Meloche, D., & Cohen, S. R. (2005). Parental perspectives on hospital staff members' acts of kindness and commemoration after a child's death. *Pediatrics, 116*(4), 884–890.

Macpherson, C. F. (2008). Peer-supported storytelling for grieving pediatric oncology nurses. *Journal of Pediatric Oncology Nursing, 25*(3), 148–163. http://dx.doi.org/10.1177/1043454208317236.

Mendes, A. (2014). Caring inside the lines: connecting within professional boundaries. *British Journal of Nursing, 23*(19), 1041. http://dx.doi.org/10.12968/bjon.2014.23.19.1041.

Meyer, R. M. L., Li, A., Klaristenfeld, J., & Gold, J. I. (2015). Pediatric novice nurses: examining compassion fatigue as a mediator between stress exposure and compassion satisfaction, burnout, and job satisfaction. *Journal of Pediatric Nursing, 30*(1), 174–183. http://dx.doi.org/10.1016/j.pedn.2013.12.008.

Milton, C. L. (2008). Boundaries: Ethical implications for what it means to be therapeutic in the Nurse-Person relationship. *Nursing Science Quarterly, 21*(1), 18–21. http://dx.doi.org/10.1177/0894318407310755.

National Council of State Boards of Nursing (2014). *A nurse's guide to professional boundaries* Retrieved from https://www.ncsbn.org/ProfessionalBoundaries_Complete.pdf.

Olson, M. S., Hinds, P. S., Euell, K., Quargnenti, A., Milligan, M., Foppiano, P., & Powell, B. (1998). Peak and nadir experiences and their consequences described by pediatric oncology nurses. *Journal of Pediatric Oncology Nursing, 15*(1), 13–36. http://dx.doi.org/10.1177/104345429801500103.

Papadatou, D., & Bellali, T. (2002). Greek nurse and physician grief as a result of caring for children dying of cancer. *Pediatric Nursing, 28*(4), 345–364 (311p).

Papadatou, D., Martinson, I. M., & Chung, P. M. (2001). Caring for dying children: a comparative study of nurses' experiences in Greece and Hong Kong. *Cancer Nursing, 24*(5), 402–412 (411p).

Pate, M. F., & Barshay, C. (2012). Maintaining professional boundaries in the pediatric intensive care unit. *AACN Advanced Critical Care, 23*(3), 242–245. http://dx.doi.org/10.1097/NCI.0b013e31824c98cd.

Polit, D. F., & Beck, C. T. (2016). *Nursing research: generating and assessing evidence for nursing practice.* Philadelphia: Wolters Kluwer Health.

Price, J., Jordan, J., Prior, L., & Parkes, J. (2011). Living through the death of a child: a qualitative study of bereaved parents' experiences. *International Journal of Nursing Studies, 48*(11), 1384–1392. http://dx.doi.org/10.1016/j.ijnurstu.2011.05.006

Rashotte, J., Fothergill-Bourbonnais, F., & Chamberlain, M. (1997). Pediatric intensive care nurses and their grief experiences: a phenomenological study. *Heart & Lung, 26*(5), 372–386 (315p).

Reid, F. (2013). Grief and the experiences of nurses providing palliative care to children and young people at home. *Nursing Children & Young People, 25*(9), 31–36. http://dx.doi.org/10.7748/ncyp2013.11.25.9.31.e366 36p.

Roberts, J., Fenton, G., & Barnard, M. (2015). Developing effective therapeutic relationships with children, young people and their families. *Nursing Children & Young People, 27*(4), 30–35. http://dx.doi.org/10.7748/ncyp.27.4.30.e566 36p.

Rushton, C. H., Reder, E., Hall, B., Comello, K., Sellers, D. E., & Hutton, N. (2006). Interdisciplinary interventions to improve pediatric palliative care and reduce health care professional suffering. *Journal of Palliative Medicine, 9*(4), 922–933 (912p).

Rushton, C. H., Kaszniak, A. W., & Halifax, J. S. (2013). A framework for understanding moral distress among palliative care clinicians. *Journal of Palliative Medicine, 16*(9), 1074–1079. http://dx.doi.org/10.1089/jpm.2012.0490.

Stayer, D. (2016). Living with dying in the pediatric intensive care unit: a nursing perspective. *American Journal of Critical Care, 25*(4), 350–356. http://dx.doi.org/10.4037/ajcc2016251.

Stevenson, M., Achille, M., & Lugasi, T. (2013). Pediatric palliative care in Canada and the United States: a qualitative metasummary of the needs of patients and families. *Journal of Palliative Medicine, 16*(5), 566–577. http://dx.doi.org/10.1089/jpm.2011.0076 512p.

The Initiative for Pediatric Palliative Care (2014). IPPC Curriculum. Retrieved from http://www.ippcweb.org/curriculum.htm.

Thompson, C. (2007). Being clear about professional boundaries. *Kai Tiaki Nursing New Zealand, 13*(8), 29.

Tong, A., Sainsbury, P., & Craig, J. (2007). Consolidated criteria for reporting qualitative research (COREQ): a 32-item checklist for interviews and focus groups. *International Journal for Quality in Health Care, 19*(6), 349–357. http://dx.doi.org/10.1093/intqhc/mzm042.

Totka, J. P. (1996). Exploring the boundaries of pediatric practice: nurse stories related to relationships. *Pediatric Nursing, 22*(3), 191–196.

Trotochaud, K., Coleman, J. R., Krawiecki, N., & McCracken, C. (2015). Moral distress in pediatric healthcare providers. *Journal of Pediatric Nursing, 30*(6), 908–914. http://dx.doi.org/10.1016/j.pedn.2015.03.001 907p.

Weidner, N. J., Cameron, M., Lee, R. C., McBride, J., Mathias, E. J., & Byczkowski, T. L. (2011). End-of-life care for the dying child: what matters most to parents. *Journal of Palliative Care, 27*(4), 279–286.

Wright, L. D. (2006). Violating professional boundaries. *Nursing, 36*(3), 52–54.

Yam, B. M. C., Rossiter, J. C., & Cheung, K. Y. S. (2001). Caring for dying infants: experiences of neonatal intensive care nurses in Hong Kong. *Journal of Clinical Nursing, 10*(5), 651–659. http://dx.doi.org/10.1046/j.1365-2702.2001.00532.x 659p.

Zander, M., Hutton, A., & King, L. (2010). Coping and resilience factors in pediatric oncology nurses. *Journal of Pediatric Oncology Nursing, 27*(2), 94–108. http://dx.doi.org/10.1177/1043454209350154.

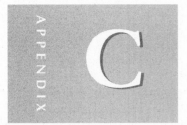

M. Cecilia Wendler, Katherine Smith, Wanda Ellenburg, Rita Gill, Lea Anderson and Kim Spiegel-Thayer Study

CrossMark

"To See With My Own Eyes": Experiences of Family Visits During Phase 1 Recovery

M. Cecilia Wendler, PhD, RN, CCRN-K, NE-BC, Katherine Smith, RN, MSN, FNP,
Wanda Ellenburg, RN, MAN/MHA, CPAN, Rita Gill, RN, BSN, Lea Anderson, RN, BSN,
Kim Spiegel-Thayer, RN, BSN

Purpose: *Long separations are a characteristic of the day of surgery, keeping patients and their family members waiting and apart. At a time of high vulnerability, these separations can cause anxiety and worry. The purpose of this study was to identify the outcomes and experiences of patients and family members who engaged in a 5- to 10-minute supervised family visit during phase I postanesthesia recovery.*
Design: *This was a descriptive, single-group, mixed-methods study.*
Methods: *Quantitative data, gathered on the day of surgery, was obtained from patients (vital signs, state anxiety scores) and their designated family members (state anxiety scores); satisfaction with the visit was also measured. An optional second, qualitative phase included a semi-structured interview examining the remembered experiences of patients and family members.*
Finding: *A statistically significant drop in state anxiety was discovered after the visit, and satisfaction with the visit was exceedingly high. Qualitatively, patients and family members described their overwhelming relief to be able "to see with my own eyes" how well each was doing.*
Conclusions: *This study supports that family visits in the postanesthesia care unit are safe and profoundly important as an independent nursing intervention. Recommendations include implementation of family visits during postanesthesia care unit recovery for all patients and family members who desire them.*
Keywords: PACU, family visitation, postanesthesia recovery.
© 2016 by American Society of PeriAnesthesia Nurses

M. Cecilia Wendler, PhD, RN, CCRN-K, NE-BC, Director, Nursing Research and Academic Partnerships, Memorial Medical Center, Springfield, IL; Katherine Smith, RN, MSN, FNP, Former Charge RN and Clinical Nurse II, PACU, Memorial Medical Center, Springfield, IL; Wanda Ellenburg, RN, MAN/MHA, CPAN, Former Nurse Manager, PACU, Memorial Medical Center, Springfield, IL; Rita Gill, RN, BSN, Clinical Nurse III, PACU, Springfield, IL; Lea Anderson, RN, BSN, Clinical Nurse II, Springfield, IL; and Kim Spiegel-Thayer, RN, BSN, Former: Clinical Nurse II, PACU, Springfield, IL.
Conflict of interest: None to report.
Address correspondence to M. Cecilia Wendler, Nursing Research and Academic Partnerships, Memorial Medical Center, 701 N. First Street, Mail Code 11, Springfield, IL 62781-0001; e-mail address: wendler.cecilia@mhsil.com.

© 2016 by American Society of PeriAnesthesia Nurses
1089-9472/$36.00
http://dx.doi.org/10.1016/j.jopan.2015.03.015

LESS THAN 20% OF AMERICAN postanesthesia care units (PACUs) allow family visitation in the first hour after surgery despite strong advocacy by researchers and the American Society of PeriAnesthesia Nurses for patient/family visits.[1-3] Restricting visitation during the recovery phase is in conflict with the needs of family members who, in one study, identified the need to visit a family member soon after surgery as one of their top two needs.[4] Indeed, families "have consistently indicated strong support for visitation ... [because of their need to know] that their loved one is safe and comfortable."[1]

Despite the evidence that supports PACU visitation,[2] including the safety and efficacy of such visits, family visits were not routine at this 500-bed Magnet-designated facility in the Midwest. Anecdotally, the nursing staff wondered: Were phase 1 visits safe for the patient and family member? And would these visits reduce anxiety and increase satisfaction with care? The purpose of this study was to close the research-practice gap and identify the outcomes and experiences of patients and family members who engaged in a 5- to 10-minute supervised family visit during phase I postanesthesia recovery.

Background

The usual surgical experience for patients in American hospitals means long separations from families and waiting while preparing for the procedure, during the procedure, and during recovery. In this hospital, patients and family members may be separated from one to several hours, a time filled with stress. Researchers have found that separation of patients from their loved ones during the surgical process involves feelings of anxiety, fear, hopelessness, and helplessness, and family members described their wait as distressing, horrible, frustrating, stressful, brutal, and difficult.[5,6] Researchers found that waiting family members endeavored to maintain a balance between negative and positive feelings from the time of separation to the time of reunion after surgery.[6]

A solution to these negative experiences might be early family visitation postoperatively, preferably within the first hour.[2] Smykowski and Rodriguez[7] found that family visitation during the PACU stay improved overall patient and family satisfaction. Farber[8] suggested that "allowing patients and their family members to be connected throughout the perioperative experience is a powerful nursing intervention." William Johnson, system director for the patient experience in this study hospital (e-mail communication, September 2011), supported this notion:

> Bringing the family bedside with their loved one in the PACU provides the unique opportunity of not only providing information but also allows the family to see, speak to and touch their loved one. This brief but critically important patient and family focused moment along their journey strongly influences overall satisfaction and perceived quality of care.

While discussing potential family visits with staff in this hospital, nurses wondered if such visits were safe for patients and their family members, and concerns arose about what *might* happen during the visit. These concerns included potential harm to the patients through disrupting vital signs (VSs) or untoward family responses, such as fainting or nausea/vomiting. Concerns about patient privacy were also raised. None of these concerns were found in the literature; however, the literature did reveal benefits of early family visits.[2] This research study was specifically designed to address staff nurse questions and provide them with an experience of family visitation under controlled circumstances to evaluate the feasibility and patient/family outcomes of such visits.

Purpose

The purpose of this study was to discover and describe the experiences of total joint replacement patients and their family members who participated in a brief family visit during phase 1 recovery. Using a descriptive and mixed-methods design,[9] we chose a 5- to 10-minute supervised phase 1 family visit and selected patient and family outcomes for patients (n = 62 dyads) undergoing total hip and knee replacement with spinal anesthesia, along with their selected family members. Spinal anesthesia patients were chosen because of their prolonged spinal anesthesia recovery process without the need for intubation/extubation; these patients are alert on arrival in the PACU and usually stay between 90 and 120 minutes. The three research questions were as follows:

1. What is the description of phase 1 family visit related to *patients'* state anxiety, mean blood pressure, and heart rate (HR) over time and satisfaction with the visit?
2. What is the description of phase 1 family visit related to *family members'* state anxiety and satisfaction with the visit?
3. What is the description of what it is like for both patients and family members who experience phase 1 family visit in the PACU?

Review of the Literature

Patient and Family State Anxiety

DeLeskey[3] found that "patients in the PACU are in a highly dependent and vulnerable state." In the presence of danger, anxiety helps the individual avoid coping.[10] State anxiety is an emotional state consisting of "unpleasant, consciously perceived feeling of tension, apprehension, nervousness, and worry, with associated activation or arousal of the autonomic nervous system,"[10] a notion supported by others.[11] Poole[12] found a decline in mean state anxiety scores from previsit to postvisit in patients randomized to receive a PACU family visit. In fact, family visitation in the PACU reduced anxiety of patients and family members in several studies.[1,7,13,14]

Family Waiting

Smykowski and Rodriguez[7] stated that family members play an integral role in family member hospitalization and are truly an expansion of the patient. Waiting is particularly stressful for the family.[5,6,15,16] Phase 1 PACU family visits reduced family anxiety[1] related to separation that occurs frequently during hospitalization.[17]

Patient and Family Satisfaction With Visit

Farber[8] stated that "allowing patients and their family members to be connected throughout the perioperative experience is a powerful nursing intervention and one that nurses in the PACU can implement to make every patient's surgical experience a positive one." Family visitation in the PACU improved overall patient and family satisfaction,[7] and Cunningham et al[18] argued that in a competitive health care market, this is important to health care providers. This idea is strongly supported by others.[8,19-22] Trimm and Sanford[6] found that family members, who were invited into the PACU for a visit and see and touch their loved ones as well as ask questions and talk to the nurse, realigned their thoughts and feelings into a more balanced state,[19] an idea in harmony with adaptation.[23]

Vital Signs

VSs, measured in this study as mean arterial blood pressure (MAP) and HR, are key indicators of body stress, especially during phase 1 recovery. VS variation by this nursing staff was addressed by VS monitoring at baseline, in the middle of the visit, and at the end of the visit, using the Dräger Infinity Delta monitor (Delta series, with software VF9; Drager Medical Systems, Inc., Telford, PA.). This device has a "motion-tolerant ... algorithm which uses a step-deflation method"[24] to obtain a blood pressure reading.

Theoretical Framework

The theoretical underpinning of this study is Roy's adaptation model.[23] This theory posits that the patient is a biopsychosocial being constantly in interaction with the environment. Stress is encountered in everyday life and extraordinary circumstances, and the human being responds to these stimuli in complex ways. One of the goals of nursing using Roy's framework is the support of successful coping by the patient as she or he becomes integrated and whole.

In this approach, the overall surgical experience/event is seen as the focal stimuli[23] for both the patient and the family member, and the relationship between and among family members is the context encountered by the patient and family as an extraordinary set of stressors. From anesthesia to the surgery to the separation caused by the focal stimuli, all aspects are at play within the PACU environment. Residual stimuli, reflected in past health care experience memories, as well as successful—or unsuccessful—prior coping for the family as a whole, mediate the situation. Total separation among family members at a time of extraordinary stress is unusual in American society,[23] and enforcement of this separation during phase 1 recovery is seen as a major contextual stimuli.

The family visit as a nursing intervention in this study is specifically designed to mitigate the separation contextual stimulus and intended to mitigate incomplete coping by providing a family visit that assists cognitive-emotive and regulator subsystems. The interdependence mode, in which "affectional needs are met ... provide[s] the individual with a feeling of security in being nurtured ... in receiving growth-producing care and attention."[17] Reducing the stress response of both the patient and the family member, here expressed as state anxiety, is the specific goal of the family visit intervention.

Methods

This descriptive, single-group, and mixed-methods study[9] was approved by the community institutional review board before the onset of the study. This complimentary mixed-methods approach was chosen to "measure overlapping ... but different facets of a phenomenon, yielding an enriched, elaborated understanding."[9(p258)] Quantitative data were obtained to determine the feasibility, safety, and selected outcomes of a 5- to 10-minute family visit during phase 1 recovery. Specifically, patients were observed for untoward responses, such as a change in VSs, whereas family members were observed for any incidence of nausea, fainting, or other problem not yet identified in the literature. Satisfaction with the visit for both the patient and the family member was also measured quantitatively.

Qualitative data were gathered to provide a more holistic picture of the experience of a family visit during phase 1 anesthesia recovery for both the patient and the family member. Qualitative data provided insight into the meaning of the visit; we were unable to find any study that had reported a comprehensive description of the experience of a family visit using qualitative approaches.

The study occurred in two phases: phase 1, on the day of surgery, within the hospital, where baseline data were gathered and the visit took place (n = 62 patients and family members) and phase 2 (optional; patients and families opted in following completion of phase 1) took place at a time and place of convenience, via telephone (n = 38 patients and family members), within 2 to 14 days of discharge from the hospital, to allow ample time for patients to be contacted, to accommodate if they had a brief and required nursing home stay before home discharge. Figure 1 illustrates the flow of the patients and family members through the study.

Sample

Using a convenience sample for study feasibility, a total of 62 dyads, consisting of a patient and his or her selected family member, served as subjects in the study. Patients 18 years and older underwent planned hip or knee replacement with spinal anesthesia. A family member was defined as any person (18 years and older) the patient designated. All patients/family members were recruited after attendance at a preoperative educational session, which occurred 1 to 2 weeks before the scheduled surgery. Patients were excluded from the study if they required general anesthesia, if they did not have a designated family member present for the visit, if they did not want the visit, or if they

were not willing to complete the consenting process.

Recruitment

Subjects were recruited through the JointWorks educational program, an optional 2-hour educational program that specifically teaches joint replacement patients and their family members what to expect before, during, immediately after, and long term as a result of the procedure. All orthopaedic surgeons serving this Magnet hospital strongly encourage their patients and a loved one to attend the JointWorks program before the day of the surgery; approximately half do so. This small class is usually attended within 1 to 2 weeks before surgery. Researchers offered the invitation to participate after the end of the educational portion of the program. In all cases, consent was completed before the day of the surgery.

Setting

The first phase of the study took place in a busy 19-bed PACU, where more than 1,200 hip and knee replacement surgeries were completed in 2011, in level 1 trauma, academically affiliated 500-bed Magnet hospital in the Midwest. Family visits were only rarely allowed in this PACU before the onset of the study. The PACU was designed over 4 decades ago, with placement of stretchers close together in recovery bays, with curtains separating the stretchers. Curtains were used to maintain privacy of patients during family visits. Data collection occurred at the patient's bedside while the staff nurse responsible for the patient was nearby. The setting also included a remodeled family waiting area just outside the PACU doors and staffed by hospital volunteers.

Research assistants who performed the data collection were highly experienced PACU registered nurses (RNs), educated in protocol implementation, and who accompanied the family member during the visit. Thus, the care nurse maintained responsibility for the patient, whereas the PACU RN research assistant maintained responsibility for the family member, in case of any untoward responses during the visit.

Baseline data for the first part of the study were gathered from both the patient and the family

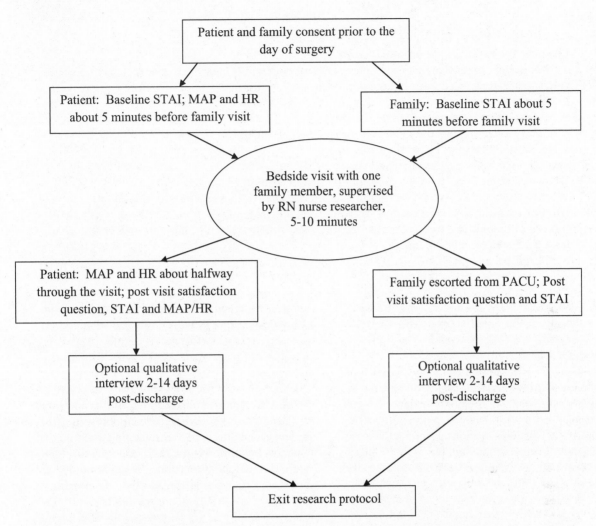

Figure 1. Flow of the subjects through the study. STAI, Spielberger State-Trait Anxiety Inventory; PACU, postanesthesia care unit; MAP, mean arterial pressure; HR, heart rate. Satisfaction question: "On a scale of 0-4 with 0 being 'no satisfaction' and 4 being 'the most satisfied I can be,' how satisfied were you with the family visit?"

members after the end of the surgery and after the surgeon had given a verbal report of surgery to waiting family members. Thus, at baseline, all patients had arrived safely in the PACU after their planned procedures, and family members were approached for baseline data while in the waiting room after hearing from the physician that the surgery was over. Family members were then escorted to the nearby family conferencing room in the surgical waiting area for baseline data collection before the planned visit.

The second phase of the study occurred after the patient had been discharged home; almost all interviews included both the patient and the designated family member responding to the semistructured interview questions at the same time, via telephone, at a time of convenience for both the patient and the family member. All interviews were scheduled in advance as appointments, and all were completed by a single and skilled qualitative researcher who interviewed the participants via telephone in a private office; these were digitally recorded with the subjects' permission. Semistructured interview questions appear in Box 1.

Measurement of Study Outcomes

Outcomes of interest were state anxiety and satisfaction with the visit for both the patients and their designated family members. Further, VS stability was an outcome for patients.

Box 1. Qualitative semistructured interview questions

1. It is okay for me to record our interview?
2. As best as you can recall, what was it like to wait for your family member to complete the surgery?
3. What was it like to wait during the postanesthesia care unit (PACU) period before you saw your family member?
4. What was it like to wait after the PACU visit?
5. What was it like to have the family visit while the patient was in the PACU?
6. What did you like most about the family visit?
7. What did you dislike about the family visit?
8. What would you recommend to us about the family visit?
9. What would you like to tell us about the family visit that we have forgotten to ask you?
10. *Quantitative satisfaction question*: Looking back on the family visit, on a scale of 0 to 4, with 0 being "not at all satisfied" and 4 being "the most satisfied I can be," how satisfied were you with the family visit in the PACU?

STATE ANXIETY. State anxiety was measured in this study using the Spielberger State-Trait Anxiety Inventory (STAI), a valid and reliable tool.[10,25] It has been developed for all ages, translated into several languages, and is written at the fourth-grade reading level. It consists of 20 questions, and answers are provided on a Likert scale of 1 to 4, with a range of possible scores being 20 to 80. Scores of 20 to 39 are considered of low state anxiety, 40 to 59 of moderate state anxiety, and 60 to 80 of high state anxiety.[10] The tool is widely reported to be valid and reliable.[10,16] State anxiety was measured at baseline, with the patient in the PACU and family member in the conference room immediately before the family visit, and again, immediately after the visit. Patients and family members served as their own controls.

PATIENT AND FAMILY SATISFACTION. Patient and family satisfaction is an important outcome[20] and was measured using a simple and unidimensional question, which was asked on the day of the visit and again, via telephone, during the optional follow-up interview. The question was provided verbally: "On a scale of 0-4, with zero meaning 'not at all satisfied' and four meaning 'the most satisfied I can be,' how satisfied were you with your family visit" [in the PACU]?

Patient and family satisfaction was also measured immediately after the visit but not while in each others' presence. The second measure of patient/family satisfaction was obtained during the follow-up interview; most of the patients and family members were interviewed together; therefore, these postdischarge measures of satisfaction were each heard at the same time as the interviewer.

VITAL SIGNS. VSs are monitored routinely during the PACU phase 1 recovery period in this setting using the Dräger Infinity Delta vital signs monitor. This has a "motion-tolerant ... algorithm which uses a step-deflation method."[24] The monitors are placed on a calibrated simulator by the biomedical engineer for annually ensuring validity and reliability of results as recommended by the manufacturer, as described by a company representative, K. Rosholt, in an e-mail communication (April 2012).

Because there were concerns that family visits could disrupt patients' VSs, MAP and HR were monitored and recorded before, during, and after the visit. For evaluation of MAP and HR, patients served as their own controls.

At the end of the postvisit data collection, patients and family members were asked, "May we contact you for the optional interview after you get home from the hospital?" Subjects self-selected into the optional phase 2 portion of the study by affirming "yes;" they were then contacted via telephone for an appointment for the interview between 2 and 14 days after discharge to home, either directly from the hospital or after a shore acute rehabilitation stay in a skilled nursing facility.

Data Analysis

Quantitative

Descriptive statistics were used to describe the sample. State anxiety was evaluated using repeated-measures *t* tests. VSs were evaluating using repeated-measures analysis of variance, isolating three sets of VSs for the patients; baseline, approximate midvisit, and end of the visit. State anxiety was evaluated using repeated-measures *t* tests.

Qualitative

Qualitative data analysis processes were carefully designed, with triangulation of researchers who were fully immersed in the data. Open coding methodology[26] using paper and pencil was used to evaluate the 38 interviews of patients and family members that were transcribed verbatim.

Qualitative data analysis requires a careful consideration of all words, phrases, stories, and ideas of the participants. Open coding allows researchers to generate many codes.[27] Data were first reduced using a by-hand open coding methodology, in which researchers "stay close to the data" using in vivo codes,[26] which involves using actual quotes from the participants for as long as possible during repeated data reduction. In this study, all researchers evaluated a single case (no. 7), which was discussed together until we reached approximately >90% agreement, ensuring inter-rater consistency of data analysis. This case served as a training case for the members of the research team who had not completed this process before.

The remainders of the transcripts were divided among five of the six researchers with the research consultant (MCW) evaluating all cases; therefore, each transcript was evaluated by at least two researchers. As data analysis proceeded, each research team member met with the experienced qualitative researcher to discuss data reduction, at all times preserving the voice and words of the patient or the family member. Each dyad of researchers discussed the data and coding, until agreement was reached. Using constant comparison,[26] codes were collapsed until data saturation occurred, yielding a total of 243 secondary codes.

In the final data reduction, all 243 secondary codes were alphabetized by first word or phrase and prepared in a large print. The final data reduction was also completed by hand. This was done in a single immersion day (Figures 2 and 3) with all members of the team present, discussing each of the category examples until agreement was arrived at, and a statement or category was placed. All data extracted were connected to the original transcript by case number, and whenever it was unclear which category a particular statement belonged to, the team returned to the original transcript to verify that the patient and/or family member's statement was preserved. In this way, the audit trail[27] was maintained.

The final data reduction resulted in 14 categories. As the categories emerged from the data, the overarching metatheme was identified and verified by all members of the research team. All documents related to data reduction were retained and form the audit trail.

The rigor of this qualitative study was assured as credibility, transferability, dependability, and confirmability are verifiable.[26] Credibility was supported through triangulation of researchers and maintaining fidelity to the participants' own words. Transferability was demonstrated when research results were presented to numerous audiences of PACU nurses, who expressed verbally their ability to implement similar changes in their own units. Dependability occurred through a careful description of the processes used to evaluate the quantitative and qualitative data. Confirmability was supported in the research results of the

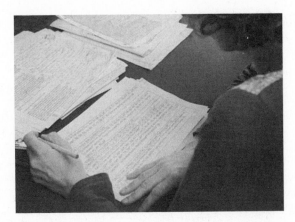

Figure 2.   Qualitative data analysis. This figure is available in color online at www.jopan.org.

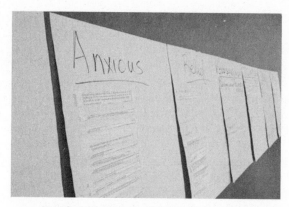

Figure 3. Data reduction into categories. This figure is available in color online at www.jopan.org.

participants' own words. Therefore, the study was rigorous.[26]

Results

Demographics

As demonstrated in Table 1, the analyzed data were derived from 62 dyads with each composed of a patient and his or her designated family member. There were three subject exclusions, two from patient and one from family member participants. Demographics revealed that patients and family members were similar to the general population of joint replacement patients at this hospital, comprising of primarily females (patient = 66% and family member = 69%) and Caucasian (patient = 95% and family member = 92%). The mean age of the patients was 62.9 (range, 30 to 87) and family members was 58.3 (range, 31 to 85).

Phase I: STAI

Cronbach's alpha,[26] which evaluates the internal consistency of a tool, was 0.92, supporting the tool's reliability[25,28] in this study. Repeated-samples *t* tests were used to calculate the state

Table 1. Demographics (n = 62)

	Age (M/SD)	Race, % White/ Minority	Gender, % Men/ Women
Patient	62.9/10.77	95.2/4.8	33.9/66.1
Family member	58.8/12.77	91.9/6.4	40.3/58.1

M, mean; SD, standard deviation.
Not all participants indicated race/gender.

Table 2. State-Trait Anxiety Inventory (State Version)

	Time 1	Time 2		
	(M/SD)		*T*	*P*
Patient	28.31/7.94	25.26/7.67	5.63	< .001
Family member	29.66/10.21	25.44/7.66	5.40	< .001

M, mean; SD, standard deviation.

anxiety responses of patients and their family members. Table 2 illustrates the patients' and family members' mean STAI before and after the visit, indicating a clinically and statistically significant reduction in state anxiety after the visit (*P* < .001).

Phase I: Physiologic Responses

Mean blood pressure and HR were obtained at three intervals during the protocol and evaluated using repeated-measures analysis of variance. As shown in Table 3, the results were nonsignificant.

Phase II: Qualitative Results

The final data reduction resulted in identification of 14 categories, which described the content, and the overarching theme emerged. Only seven secondary codes did not fit within the final structure; these were set aside and not included in the final analysis. Categories with examples from the data that support the categories appear in Table 4.

Patient Satisfaction

Patient satisfaction was reported by the patient and family member both directly following the family (n = 62) and at the end of the optional phase II interview. Table 5 demonstrates these results.

Discussion

The short family visit during phase 1 recovery "is a powerful nursing intervention"[8] and was tested in this innovative, complimentary, and mixed-methods study.[9] The goal was to more fully understand the patient and family experience of a family visit after joint replacement surgery under spinal anesthesia. Results supported past studies[1,7,13,14] that a supervised 5- to 10-minute[11] visit significantly and substantially reduced the state anxiety

Table 3. Patient MBP and HR (Repeated-Measures ANOVA Using Wilks' Lambda)

	Baseline	Beginning of Visit	End of Visit		
	(M/SD)			F	P
MBP	90.52/13.84	90.02/13.17	89.37/1,356	(2, 59) = 0.56	.573
HR	66.11/9.01	66.69/9.32	60.09/11.24	(2, 59) = 0.356	.702

MBP, mean blood pressure; HR, heart rate; ANOVA, analysis of variance; M, mean; SD, standard deviation.

of both the patient and the designated family member ($P < .001$) at a time of high vulnerability[13]; with the focal stimuli and the immediacy of the environment that can produce stress.[23] Roy adaptation theory[23] would predict that a family visit would modulate the stress of waiting after surgery through coping, and this, in fact, was the result.[23] Prior work of several researchers who have also tested a family visit under a variety of surgical situations[1,7,14] supports this notion.

Patelarou et al[29] recently reported results that conflict with the present study. In a study of Greek patients and their related family members, they concluded that there was no clinically significant reduction in state anxiety when family visits were allowed, despite a strong statistical reduction reported. This study did not discuss preoperative educational efforts. Education may have helped to prevent the high levels of anxiety reported in the study by Patelarou et al.[29] Secondarily, Patelarou et al[29] allowed a wide variety of surgical procedure patients into their study; the present study controlled for this variability. Third, the present study included patients experiencing spinal anesthesia, whereas the Greek study did not define anesthesia status. Also, there may have been cultural differences between US and Greek patients and family members when encountering the surgical experience.

At the outset of the study, the staff of this PACU listed several concerns that were more myth than truth; such concerns did not appear in the literature. One myth held by the staff was that patients or family members might somehow be harmed because of the family visit; the visit itself might be unsafe. For this reason, the present study examined patient VSs, and family member visits were supervised so that patients were cared for by the PACU staff nurse and family members could have been cared for by the research nurse if required.

However, no untoward effect to either patient or family members occurred. VSs of patients remained unchanged during and after the family visit, and no family member experienced any untoward response (fainting, nausea, or emotional outburst) during the study. Another stated worry was that privacy and confidentiality could not be maintained and that there would be interruptions in care flow. However, informal observation during the study revealed that patients and family members visiting were respectful of the need for privacy of others, and care flow was not disrupted. Thus, these common myths were dispelled, and anecdotal comments by staff indicate their comfort with activities related to the family visit; feasibility of the visits in this PACU was demonstrated.

The study presented two opportunities to measure patient and family satisfaction: First, on the day of the surgery just after the visit (n = 62 dyads) and again, after discharge, for those participating in the optional interview. The mean of the first assessment was exceedingly high, measuring 3.95 of a possible 4 for patients and 3.97 for family members. This indicates a very high level of patient and family satisfaction and supports the same conclusion of Smykowski and Rodriguez.[7] This result persisted over time and became a lasting memory of satisfaction: Patients (n = 36) reported an average of 3.92 of 4 during the follow-up interview, whereas 38 family members reported an average of 3.92 of 4. A preponderance of high scores on the satisfaction scale may indicate a ceiling effect of the unidimensional tool used to measure satisfaction and may be a limitation of the study.

Qualitative results revealed rich data about the experience of a short family visit. Patients and their family members discussed in depth their sense of appreciation for the opportunity to see their family member soon after surgery. Anticipation of the visit prevented some experiences of anxiety, and

Appendix C

Table 4. Qualitative Results: Categories With Supporting Codes

Category	Selected Examples [Supporting Case Numbers]
Anticipation	"Just knowing that [family member] was going to come back there early relaxed me" [75]
	Anticipated [visit] with excitement [09, 43]
	Really wanted to see [patient] [39, 43]
Anxiety	"very anxious" [03, 06, 07, 08, 09, 14, 20, 23, 36, 39, 43, 46, 50, 58, 59, 64, 65, 73, 77, 80]
	"anxious to see how [pt] was doing" [07, 25, 27, 33, 39, 43, 60]
	"Nervous" [08, 09, 20, 23, 39, 46]
Caring	"Just knowing how much they cared" [68]
	To see patient being cared for/to be cared for [07, 09, 10, 20, 41, 65]
Communication	"to be kept informed [10, 43, 64]; to know what was going on [09, 13, 45, 50, 53, 57, 58, 60, 64, 65, 73, 74]
	Laughed and joked during the visit [06, 25, 27, 38, 43, 50, 57, 59, 69, 73, 76]
	Touching [02, 03, 06, 07, 08, 09, 10, 14, 20, 22, 23, 33, 36, 39, 41, 50, 65, 75]
Glad surgery is over	"We are over the slump of [surgery and anesthesia] [06, 25, 33, 37, 39, 41, 43, 45, 48, 52, 58, 60, 64, 73, 74, 80]
	"If they [allowed family visits], then everything was OK" [45, 48]
Hospitality	Volunteers [in the waiting area] helpful, informative [48, 58, 60, 65, 68, 69]
	PACU [nurses] "did not hurry visit" [60]
Long-term relationships	"S/he's been my partner a long time" [43]; "the love of my life [33, 39]
	"We have a special relationship" [68, 69]
	Patient/family watching out for each other [73]
PACU characteristics	"calm atmosphere" [39, 68]; "energy really nice" [33, 60]
	Busy [27, 28, 43, 45, 74]
	Afraid of disrupting equipment or injuring patient [23, 28, 41]
Patient experiences	"Confusion; muddled; groggy" [13, 22, 23, 27, 33, 36, 39, 43, 48, 49, 50, 57, 64, 65, 68, 73, 74, 75, 76, 77, 80]
	"Had a kind of out of body experience" [64, 77]
	"It's a big deal [family] was allowed [to visit] [41]
Presence	"To be there" [08, 22, 23, 65]
	"Presence" [39, 43, 45, 50]
	To have an advocate … right there … accessible [10] "for support and encouragement" [65]
Relief	"Overwhelming relief" [46, 49, 64]; relief [03, 06, 14, 20, 22, 23, 25, 36, 38, 41, 43, 45, 48, 50, 58, 64, 65, 73]
	Reassure/reassurance [02, 03, 06, 07, 09, 10, 14, 28, 36, 37, 38, 39, 45, 49]
	To know "everything was fine … a critical thing" [22, 64, 73];
	"everything's OK" [50, 58, 60, 64, 69, 73, 75, 76, 77, 80]
"To see with my own eyes"	"To see with my own eyes [28]; "to see for myself" [13, 25, 27, 28, 33, 37, 69, 73, 74, 80]
	"When I saw him, I knew [the patient] was OK" [39, 41]; When I saw my family, I knew they were OK, too [42, 43, 45, 46, 48, 49, 53, 58, 60, 64, 65, 68]
Visit: characteristics, outcomes, and recommendations	Did not dislike anything about the visit [06, 13, 20, 23, 25, 27, 28, 33, 36, 37, 38, 41, 43, 45, 46, 48, 49, 50, 53, 57, 58, 59, 60, 68, 73, 75, 77, 80]
	Visit "a good thing" [02, 03, 07, 09, 10, 13, 14, 22, 23, 27, 28, 36, 37, 38, 43, 45, 46, 48, 49, 50, 58, 60, 64, 65, 69, 73, 75, 77];
	visit "great" [06, 41, 53, 59]
	Visit helps to get self-awareness [06, 28, 33]
	"helps to ground [patient] [58]; grounds patient quicker [06, 10, 27, 34, 36, 50, 77, 80]
	"Just what I needed" [20, 43, 50]

(Continued)

TO SEE WITH MY OWN EYES

Table 4. Continued

Category	Selected Examples [Supporting Case Numbers]
Wait: Characteristics	"Recommend [PACU nurses prepare family] for the [visiting] process" [20, 27]
	Waiting "was long" [03, 07, 08, 09, 10, 13, 33, 43, 45, 50, 64, 65, 68, 69, 73, 76, 77]
	Waiting was "just fine/ok" [02, 03, 06, 10, 14, 27, 28, 33, 36, 37, 38, 39, 41, 45, 46, 48, 49, 50, 53, 57, 59, 60, 64, 65, 68, 73, 74, 76, 80]
	[Pt has] No memory of waiting/little memory of waiting [14, 22, 23, 27, 28, 33, 36, 43, 48, 49, 50, 57, 58, 64, 68, 69, 74, 75, 76, 77, 80]

PACU, postanesthesia care unit.

the wait during and after surgery was characterized by a sense of hospitality and welcome for most. Seeing the visit as an opportunity to receive caring communication, many family members expressed relief that surgery was successfully completed. Qualitative results matched quantitative results. The visit reduced the reported anxiety of both the patient and the family member, both of whom found the visit grounding.

Although the surroundings of the PACU were sometimes unfamiliar to family members, they were most grateful for the opportunity to actually be there, providing a soothing presence for each other. It relieved the long wait for both, and for some, it asserted the centrality of their long-term relationships with each other, many openly affirming this during the interviews.

Several patients reported a sense of grogginess that lifted when the family member was either heard or seen during the visit. Remarkably, two of the patients interviewed described vivid out-of-body experiences, despite the fact that they had not undergone general anesthesia. These two patients described clearly how they hovered above their bodies, as they scanned the room from above;

seeing their loved ones approaching the cart, they both reported an immediate and physical sensation of re-entering their own bodies quickly, and then greeting their loved one when the visit commenced. We did not encounter any other reports in the literature of out-of-body experiences in the PACU.

The overarching theme, "*to see with my own eyes,*" was repeated over and over in the qualitative data, indicating its centrality as a study result. Many patients and family members expressed appreciation for the family report, but the power of being able to see, touch, kiss, and converse with family members was very important to both the patient and the family member,[4] helping to relieve the common negative experiences of waiting.[5]

Family visits during phase 1 recovery are safe and effective as an independent nursing intervention. This study adds strong evidence that affirms American Society of PeriAnesthesia Nurses's[2] recommendations that family visits be allowed for all patients who experience a stay in the PACU.

Perianesthesia Implications

This study demonstrates that brief family visits during phase 1 anesthesia recovery significantly and substantially reduces anxiety for both the patients and the family members. Implications for nursing were identified and may be appropriate for use in patient care, education, and research.

Nursing Practice

Despite staff initial resistance to this practice change,[30] the research study allowed the team to

Table 5. Satisfaction With the Visit

	End of Visit	After Hospital Discharge
	M (SD)	
Patient	3.95 (0.22); n = 62	3.92 (0.28); n = 36
Family member	3.97 (0.18); n = 61	3.92 (0.27); n = 38

M, mean; SD, standard deviation; n, number of participants.

test the feasibility and outcomes of a short visit during phase 1 recovery for patients receiving spinal anesthesia. Qualitative comments from both the patient and the family members were powerful tools to illustrate the importance and value of the family visit to staff nurses practicing in this PACU. Anecdotally, once staff nurses saw the visit was safe for both the patient and the family members, resistance to implementation diminished. Soon after completion of this study, the visiting policy (available on request) was changed to allow brief family visits for all patients who desired them.

Specific recommendations for nursing practice include the following:

- Involve staff nurses in the planned change; perhaps create a role of a staff champion for that change. If possible, have staff nurses lead the change.
- Manager and leader support for any change is critical and needed before the onset of such a planned change.
- Reward and recognize staff for implementing change early after the change and at regular intervals thereafter.

Education

Staff nurses need to be fully educated about the visiting process to provide consistent communication and structure to the visit. Patients and family members need to be prepared in advance by explaining the parameters of the visit and what to expect. This could occur in the preoperative education setting, or it can occur on the day of surgery.

Hospital volunteers played a very important role in helping the family members feel welcomed and informed in the milieu of the surgical waiting area. Therefore, volunteers also need to be educated on the structure and process of phase 1 family visits so that communication between patients, family members, staff, and volunteers can be consistent and meet set expectations.

Research

This study evaluated phase 1 family visit for patients undergoing spinal anesthesia. Further research may provide insight on the most effective time for family visits. It is unclear whether patients

undergoing general anesthesia would have different outcomes with the family visit; further research is needed to determine the safety and usefulness of family visits for these patients. In particular, families of patients who arrive in the PACU in a physiologically unstable state might require different preparation for the visit or another intervention, such as the family presence during resuscitation. These situations were not tested in this study.

It is not known if, or in what way, family visits for surgical patients might influence global outcomes such as patient satisfaction with the entire hospital experience. Further research is needed to determine the relationship, if any, of a family visit during phase 1 recovery and the patients' self-report of global satisfaction.

Limitations

Generalizability of the study is hampered by the lack of a control group, and a convenience sample was used. We did not obtain any information about those potential patients who declined inclusion into the study, so it is unknown whether there were differences between those who self-selected into the study and those who did not. Qualitative results offer a developing understanding of the experience of a family visit in the PACU. Similar PACUs, their patients and family members, might find the results useful, but because these results are context specific, careful judgment is required before findings can be transferrable to another setting.

Conclusions

Family visitation in the PACU is safe and effectively reduces anxiety; it also may improve the perception of waiting and may drive patient and family satisfaction on the day of the surgery. Although not every patient or family member may choose to visit during the early recovery period, this study, and others, provide the scientific basis for promoting family visits during phase 1 recovery. This study demonstrated the feasibility of phase 1 visits, and results provide further support for instituting family visits to reduce anxiety and enhance patient satisfaction when patients and family members agree.

TO SEE WITH MY OWN EYES

Acknowledgments

The research team thanks Hope Bridges, RN, and Gina Carnduff, RN, BSN, for early contributions to the project, as well as Gordon Forbes, PhD, for statistical consultation. The support of the project by the PACU staff at Memorial Medical Center helped to ensure its success, and the generous feedback offered by anonymous reviewers greatly improved this article. Photography credits: Bobbi Wiseman.

This project was funded in part by a generous grant from the Illinois Society of PeriAnesthesia Nurses and another by the Memorial Medical Center Foundation, Springfield, IL.

References

1. Carter A, Deselms J, Ruyle S, et al. Postanesthesia care unit visitation decreases family member anxiety. *J Perianesth Nurs.* 2012;27:3-9.

2. American Society of PeriAnesthesia Nurses. *Perianesthesia Nursing: Standards, Practice Recommendations and Interpretive Statements.* Cherry Hill, NJ: American Society of PeriAnesthesia Nurses; 2012.

3. DeLeskey K. Family visitation in the PACU: The current state of practice in the United States. *J Perianesth Nurs.* 2009; 24:81-85.

4. Cormier S, Pickett S, Gallagher J. Comparison of nurses' and family members' perceived needs during postanesthesia care unit visits. *J Post Anesth Nurs.* 1992;7:387-391.

5. Bournes D, Mitchel G. Waiting: The experience of persons in a critical care waiting room. *Res Nurs Health.* 2002;25:58-67.

6. Trimm D, Sanford J. The process of family waiting during surgery. *J Fam Nurs.* 2010;16:435-461.

7. Smykowski L, Rodriguez W. The post anesthesia care unit: A family centered approach. *J Nurs Care Qual.* 2003;18:5-15.

8. Farber J. Measuring and improving ambulatory surgery patients' satisfaction. *AORN J.* 2010;92:313-321.

9. Greene J, Caracell V, Graham W. Toward a conceptual framework for mixed-method evaluation design. *Educ Eval Policy Anal.* 1989;11:255-274.

10. Spielberger C, Summer S. State-Trait Anxiety Inventory and State-Trait Anger Expression Inventory. In: Maruish M, ed. *The Use of Psychological Testing Treatment Planning and Outcomes Assessment.* Hillsdale, NJ: Lawrence Erlbaum; 1994: 292-320.

11. Wendler MC. Effects of Tellington touch in healthy adults awaiting venipuncture. *Res Nurs Health.* 2003;26:40-52.

12. Poole E. The effects of postanesthesia care unit visits on anxiety in surgical patients. *J Post Anesth Nurs.* 1993;8:386-394.

13. Bru G, Carody S, Donohue-Sword B, Bookbinder M. Parental visitation in the postanesthesia care unit: A means to lessen anxiety. *Child Health Care.* 1993;22:217-226.

14. Roach C, Messmer P, Williams A. Hispanic parents' perspective of early PACU visitation. *J Perianesth Nurs.* 2010; 25:152-161.

15. Kutash M, Northrop L. Family member's experiences of the intensive care unit waiting room. *J Adv Nurs.* 2007;60: 384-388.

16. Muldoon M, Duniei C, Vish N, DeJohn S, Adams J. Implementation of an informational card to reduce family members' anxiety. *AORN J.* 2011;94:246-253.

17. Servonsky J, Tedrow M. Separation Anxiety and Loneliness. In: Roy C, Andrews H, eds. *The Roy Adaptation Model: The Definitive Statement.* Norwalk, CT: Appleton & Lange; 1991;405-425.

18. Cunningham M, Hanson-Heath C, Agre P. A perioperative nurse liaison program. *J Nurs Care Qual.* 2003;18:16-21.

19. DeWitt L, Albert N. Preferences of visitation in the PACU. *J Perianesth Nurs.* 2010;25:296-301.

20. Merkouris A, Ifantopoulos J, Lanara V, Lemonidou C. Patient satisfaction: A key concept for evaluating and improving nursing services. *J Nurs Manag.* 1999;7:19-28.

21. Tuller S, McCabe L, Cronenwett L, et al. Patient, visitor, and nurse evaluations of visitation for adult postanesthesia care unit patients. *J Perianesth Nurs.* 1997;12:402-412.

22. Walls M. Staff attitudes and beliefs regarding family visitation after implementation of a formal visitation policy in the PACU. *J Perianesth Nurs.* 2009;24:229-232.

23. Roy C, Andrews HA. *The Roy Adaptation Model: The Definitive Statement.* Norwalk, CT: Appleton & Lange; 1991.

24. *Dräger, Inc. Resource Manual: Monitoring and IT Solutions for Supporting Patient Safety and Care.* Telford, PA: Dräger, Inc; 2010.

25. Ramanaiah V, Franzen M, Schill T. A psychometric study of the State-Trait Anxiety Inventory. *J Pers Assess.* 1983;47: 531-535.

26. Wuest J. Grounded Theory: The Method. In: Munhall P, ed. *Nursing Research: A Qualitative Perspective*, 4th ed. Boston, MA: Jones & Bartlett; 2007:225-256.

27. Munhall P. *Nursing Research: A Qualitative Perspective*, 4th ed. Boston, MA: Jones & Bartlett; 2007.

28. Tavakol M, Dennick R. Making sense of Cronbach's alpha. *Int J Med Educ.* 2011;2:53-55.

29. Patelarou A, Melidonioti E, Sgouraki M, Karatzi M, Souvatzis X. The effect of visiting surgical patients in the postanesthesia care unit on family members' anxiety: A prospective quasi-experimental study. *J Perianesth Nurs.* 2014;29:221-229.

30. Melnyk B, Fineout-Overholt E. *Evidence-Based Practice in Nursing and Healthcare: A Guide to Best Practice.* Philadelphia, PA: Lippincott Williams & Wilkins; 2011.

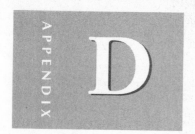

D Appraisal Guidelines

CRITICAL APPRAISAL GUIDELINES FOR A QUANTITATIVE STUDY

Step 1: Identifying the Steps or Elements of the Study; and Step 2: Determining the Study Strengths and Limitations

1. Writing quality
   a. Is the writing style of the report clear and concise with relevant terms defined?

2. Title
   a. Is the title clearly focused?
   b. Does the title include key study variables and population?
   c. Does the title indicate the type of study conducted—descriptive, correlational, quasi-experimental, or experimental—and the variables (Gray, Grove, & Sutherland, 2017; Shadish, Cook, & Campbell, 2002)?

3. Authors
   a. Do the authors have credentials such as a Doctor of Philosophy (PhD) that qualified them to conduct the presented study?
   b. Do the authors have previous research or clinical experience that qualified them to conduct the presented study?
   c. Do any of the authors have a conflict of interest related to the study, such as financial interest in the company that produced the intervention implemented in the study?

4. Abstract
   a. Is the abstract clearly presented?
   b. Does the abstract include purpose, design highlights, sample, intervention (if applicable), and key results (American Psychological Association [APA], 2010).

5. Research problem (see Chapter 5)
   a. Is a problem statement provided? If a problem statement is not provided, can you infer the problem or gap in the literature?
   b. Is the problem significant to nursing and clinical practice (Brown, 2018)?

6. Purpose
   a. State the purpose of the study.
   b. Does the purpose narrow and clarify the focus of the study (Fawcett & Garity, 2009; O'Mathúna & Fineout-Overholt, 2015)?

7. Literature review (see Chapter 6)
   a. Examine the literature review.
   b. Are most references peer-reviewed primary sources? Do the authors justify references that are not peer-reviewed primary sources?
   c. Are most of the references current (number and percentages of sources published in the last 5 and 10 years)? Are references older than 10 years, measurement or theoretical sources, landmark, seminal, or replication studies?
   d. Is the content directly related to the study concepts or variables? Are the types of sources and disciplines of the source authors appropriate for the study concepts or variables?

    e. Are the studies critically appraised and synthesized (Gray et al., 2017; Hart, 2009)? Is a clear concise summary presented of the current empirical and theoretical knowledge in the area of the study, including identifying what is known and not known (O'Mathúna & Fineout-Overholt, 2015)? Does the study address a gap in the knowledge identified in the literature review?

8. Framework or theoretical perspective (see Chapter 7)

    a. Is the framework explicitly expressed, or must you extract the framework from statements in the introduction, literature review, or other section(s) of the study?

    b. Does the framework identify, define, and describe the relationships among the concepts of interest? If a model or conceptual map of the framework is present, is it adequate to explain the phenomenon of concern (Gray et al., 2017)?

    c. How is the framework related to nursing's body of knowledge (Alligood, 2014; Smith & Liehr, 2014)?

    d. If a proposition from a theory is to be tested, is the proposition clearly identified and linked to the study hypotheses (Fawcett & Garity, 2009; Smith & Liehr, 2014)?

9. Research objectives, questions, or hypotheses (see Chapter 5)

    a. List any research objectives, questions, or hypotheses.

    b. Are the objectives, questions, or hypotheses clearly expressed and logically linked to the research purpose?

    c. Are the objectives, questions, or hypotheses logically linked to the concepts and relationships (propositions) in the framework (Chinn & Kramer, 2015; O'Mathúna & Fineout-Overholt, 2015; Smith & Liehr, 2014)?

    d. Are hypotheses stated to direct the conduct of quasi-experimental and experimental research (Shadish et al., 2002)?

10. Variables (see Chapter 5)

    a. Identify the study variables or concepts. Attributes or demographic variables should be provided. A study usually includes independent and dependent variables or research variables, but not all three types of variables.

        i. Demographic variables

        ii. Independent variables

        iii. Dependent variables

        iv. Research variables or concepts

    b. Identify the conceptual and operational definitions for independent and dependent variables.

    c. Are the variables clearly defined (conceptually and operationally) and based on previous research or theories (Chinn & Kramer, 2015; Gray et al., 2017; Smith & Liehr, 2014)?

    d. Are the variables reflective of the concepts identified in the framework?

11. Research design (see Chapter 8).

    a. Identify the specific design of the study.

    b. Does the design provide a means to examine all the objectives, questions, and hypotheses?

    c. Is the design used in the study the most appropriate design to obtain the required data (Gray et al., 2017)?

    d. Treatment

        i. Does the study include a treatment or intervention?

        ii. Is the treatment clearly described (Eymard & Altmiller, 2016)?

        iii. Is the treatment appropriate for examining the study purpose and hypotheses?

        iv. Was a protocol developed to promote consistent implementation of the treatment to ensure intervention fidelity (Eymard & Altmiller, 2016)?

        v. Did the researcher monitor implementation of the treatment to ensure consistency?

        vi. If the treatment was not consistently implemented, what might be the impact on the findings?

    e. Groups

        i. Did the study have more than one group?

        ii. If the study had more than one group, how were study participants assigned to groups?

        iii. If a treatment was implemented with more than one group, were the participants randomly assigned to the treatment group or were the treatment and comparison groups matched? Were the treatment and comparison group assignments appropriate for the purpose of the study?

        iv. If more than one group was used, did the groups appear equivalent?

f. Were pilot study findings used to design this study? If yes, briefly discuss the pilot and the changes made in this study based on the pilot (Gray et al., 2017; Shadish et al., 2002).

g. Did the researcher identify the threats to design validity (statistical conclusion validity, internal validity, construct validity, and external validity) and minimize them as much as possible (Gray et al., 2017; Shadish et al., 2002)?

12. Sample (see Chapter 9).

a. Is the sampling method probability or nonprobability? Is the specific sampling method used in the study to obtain the sample identified and appropriate (Gray et al., 2017)?

b. What are the sampling inclusion criteria and sampling exclusion criteria, and were both clearly identified and appropriate for the study (O'Mathúna & Fineout-Overholt, 2015)?

c. Is the sample size identified (Aberson, 2010)?

d. Is the refusal or acceptance rate identified? Is the sample attrition or retention rate addressed? Are reasons provided for the refusal and attrition rates?

e. Is a power analysis reported? Was the sample size appropriate, as indicated by the power analysis? If groups were included in the study, is the sample size for each group equal and appropriate (Grove & Cipher, 2017)?

f. Is the sampling process adequate to achieve a representative sample? Is the sample representative of the accessible and target populations?

g. Did the researcher(s) define the target and accessible populations for the study?

h. How was informed consent/assent obtained?

i. Was the process used for informed consent/assent appropriate for the study population?

13. Setting (see Chapter 9)

a. What is the study setting?

b. Is the setting appropriate for the study purpose?

14. Measurement (see Chapter 10)

a. Complete Table D.1 to cover essential measurement content for a study (Waltz, Strickland, & Lenz, 2017).

   i. Identify each study variable that was measured.

   ii. Identify the name and author of each measurement strategy.

   iii. Identify the type of each measurement strategy (e.g., Likert scale, visual analog scale, physiological measure, or existing database).

   iv. Identify the level of measurement (e.g., nominal, ordinal, interval, or ratio) achieved by each measurement method used in the study (Grove & Cipher, 2017).

   v. Describe the reliability of each scale for previous studies and this study. Identify the precision of each physiological measure (Bialocerkowski, Klupp, & Bragge, 2010; DeVon, et al., 2007).

   vi. Identify the validity of each scale and the accuracy of physiological measures (DeVon, et al., 2007; Ryan-Wenger, 2017).

b. Scales and questionnaires

   i. Are the instruments clearly described?

   ii. Are techniques to complete and score the instruments provided?

   iii. Did the researcher reexamine the validity and reliability of the instruments for the present sample?

   iv. If the instrument was developed for the study, is the instrument development process described (Gray et al., 2017; Waltz et al., 2017)?

Table D.1 Measurement Strategies

Variable Measured	Name of Measurement Method (Author)	Type of Measurement Method	Level of Measurement	Reliability or Precision	Validity or Accuracy

   c. Observation
      i. Is what is to be observed clearly identified and defined?
      ii. Are the techniques for recording observations described (Waltz et al., 2017)?
      iii. Is interrater reliability described?
   d. Interviews
      i. Do the interview questions address concerns expressed in the research problem?
      ii. Are the interview questions relevant for the research purpose and objectives, questions, or hypotheses (Gray et al., 2017; Waltz et al., 2017)?
   e. Physiological measures
      i. Are the physiological measures or instruments clearly described (Ryan-Wenger, 2017)? If appropriate, are the brand names of the instruments identified?
      ii. Are the accuracy, precision, and error of the physiological instruments discussed (Ryan-Wenger, 2017)?
      iii. Are the physiological measures appropriate for the research purpose and objectives, questions, or hypotheses?
      iv. Are the methods for recording data from the physiological measures clearly described? Is the recording of data consistent?
   f. Do the measurement methods selected for the study adequately measure the study variables? Should additional measurement methods have been used to improve the quality of the study outcomes (Waltz et al., 2017)?
   g. Do the measurement methods used in the study have adequate validity and reliability? What additional reliability or validity testing is needed to improve the quality of the measurement methods (Bialocerkowski et al., 2010; DeVon et al., 2007; Waltz et al., 2017)?

15. Data collection (see Chapter 10)
   a. Is the data collection process clearly described (Fawcett & Garity, 2009; Gray et al., 2017)?
   b. Do the data collected address the research objectives, questions, or hypotheses?
   c. How did the researchers ensure that the data collection process was conducted in an accurate and consistent manner?
      i. Who collected the study data?
      ii. Is the training of data collectors clearly described and adequate?
      iii. Were methods of standardization such as standardized forms or computerized data used?
   d. Was institutional review board (IRB) approval obtained before data collection?
   e. Were the data collection methods ethical?
   f. Did any adverse events occur during data collection, and were these appropriately managed?

16. Data analyses (see Chapter 11)
   a. Complete Table D.2 with the analysis techniques conducted in the study (Gray et al., 2017; Grove & Cipher, 2017; Hoare & Hoe, 2013; Plichta & Kelvin, 2013).
      i. Identify the purpose (description, relationships, or differences) for each analysis technique.
      ii. List the statistical analysis technique performed.
      iii. List the statistic.
      iv. Provide the specific results.
      v. Identify the probability (p) of the statistical significance achieved by the result.
   b. Are data analysis procedures clearly described?
   c. Do the data analysis techniques address the study purpose and the research objectives, questions, or hypotheses (Gray et al., 2017; Grove & Cipher, 2017)?

Table D.2 Statistical Analysis and Results

Purpose of Analysis	Analysis Technique	Statistic	Results	Probability (p)

d. Are data analysis procedures appropriate for the type of data collected (Grove & Cipher, 2017; Plichta & Kelvin, 2013)?

e. Did the researcher address any problem with missing data and explain how this problem was managed?

f. Statistical significance:

i. Was the level of significance or alpha identified? If yes, what was the level of significance (0.05, 0.01, or 0.001)?

ii. Is the sample size sufficient to detect significant differences if they are present?

iii. Was a power analysis conducted for nonsignificant results (Aberson, 2010)?

g. Are the results presented in an understandable way by narrative, tables, figures, or a combination of methods (APA, 2010; Grove & Cipher, 2017)?

h. Are the results interpreted appropriately?

Step 3: Evaluating the Credibility and Meaning of the Study Findings

17. Interpretation of findings

a. Are the findings consistent with previous research findings (Gray et al., 2017; O'Mathúna & Fineout-Overholt, 2015)?

b. Are findings discussed in relation to each objective, question, or hypothesis?

c. Are various explanations for significant and nonsignificant findings examined?

d. Are the findings clinically important (O'Mathúna & Fineout-Overholt, 2015)?

e. Are the findings linked to the study framework (Smith & Liehr, 2014)? If so, do the findings support the study framework?

f. What questions emerge from the findings, and does the researcher identify them?

18. Limitations

a. What study limitations did the researcher identify?

b. Does the study have limitations not identified by the researcher?

c. Could the limitations of the study have been prevented or controlled by the researcher?

19. Conclusions

a. What conclusions did the researchers identify based on their interpretation of the study findings?

b. Do the conclusions fit the findings from this study and previous studies?

c. How did the researcher generalize the findings? Did the researcher generalize the findings appropriately?

20. Nursing implications

a. What implications do the findings have for nursing practice (Melnyk, Gallagher-Ford, & Fineout-Overholt, 2017; O'Mathúna & Fineout-Overholt, 2015)?

b. Were the identified implications for practice appropriate based on the study findings and on the findings from previous research (Melnyk & Fineout-Overholt, 2015)?

21. Future research

a. What suggestions for further study were identified?

b. Were quality suggestions made for future research (O'Mathúna & Fineout-Overholt, 2015)?

c. Is the description of the study sufficiently clear for replication?

d. Did money, commitment, the researchers' expertise, availability of subjects, facilities, equipment, and/or ethics make the study unfeasible to conduct (Gray et al., 2017)?

22. Critique summary

a. Review the components of the critique you just conducted. Consider the following to formulate your critique summary.

i. Were all relevant components covered with adequate detail and clarity?

ii. What were the study's greatest strengths and greatest weaknesses?

iii. Were the rights of human subjects protected (Creswell, 2014; Gray et al., 2017)?

iv. Do you believe the study findings are valid? How much confidence can be placed in the study findings?

v. The evaluation of a research report should also include a final discussion of the quality of the report. This discussion should include an expert opinion of the study's quality and contribution to nursing knowledge and practice (Melnyk et al., 2017; O'Mathúna & Fineout-Overholt, 2015).

CRITICAL APPRAISAL GUIDELINES FOR A QUALITATIVE STUDY

Step 1: Identifying the Steps of the Research Process in Studies; and Step 2: Determining Study Strengths and Weaknesses

1. Writing quality
   a. Is the writing style of the report clear and concise with relevant terms defined?

2. Title
   a. What is the title?
   b. Is the title clearly focused, and does it include the topic and population of the study? Does the title indicate the type of study conducted—phenomenology, grounded theory, exploratory-descriptive qualitative, and ethnography (Creswell & Poth, 2018; Powers, 2015)?

3. Authors
   a. Do the authors have credentials such as a PhD degree that qualified them to conduct the presented study?
   b. Do the authors have previous research or clinical experience that qualified them to conduct the presented study?
   c. Do any of the authors have a conflict of interest, such as a financial interest related to the study?

4. Abstract
   a. Was the abstract clearly presented?
   b. Does the abstract include purpose, specific qualitative methodology, sample, and key results?

5. Research problem
   a. Is a problem statement provided? If a problem statement is not provided, can you infer the problem or gap in nursing's knowledge from the introduction and literature review?
   b. Is the problem significant to nursing and clinical practice (Cohen & Crabtree, 2008)?

6. Purpose
   a. State the purpose.
   b. Does the purpose narrow and clarify the focus of the study (Creswell, 2014; Fawcett & Garity, 2009)?

7. Literature review
   a. Are most references peer-reviewed primary sources? Do the authors justify references that are not peer-reviewed primary sources?
   b. Are the references current (number and percentage of sources in the last 5 and 10 years)? Are references older than 10 years, measurement or theoretical sources, landmark, seminal, or replication studies?
   c. Is the content directly related to the study concepts? Are the types of sources and disciplines of the source authors appropriate for the study concepts?
   d. Are the studies critically appraised and synthesized (Fawcett & Garity, 2009; Gray et al., 2017; Hart, 2009)? Is a clear concise summary presented of the current empirical and theoretical knowledge in the area of the study, including identifying what is known and not known (Gray et al., 2017)?

8. Philosophical orientation or study framework
   a. Was the philosophical orientation of the qualitative approach identified? Was a primary source for the philosophy cited (Creswell & Poth, 2018; Gray et al., 2017; Munhall, 2012)?
   b. If a framework was used, are its major concepts reflected in the questions asked during data collection and in the findings?
   c. Grounded theory
      i. Did the researcher develop a theoretical description or diagram as part of the study findings (Creswell & Poth, 2018)?
      ii. If a framework was developed from the findings (grounded theory study), is it clearly linked to the study findings?

9. Research objectives (aims) or questions
   a. Are the objectives (aims) or questions identified and clearly presented?
   b. List the provided research objectives (aims) or questions, if identified.
   c. Are the objectives or questions linked to the research purpose?

10. Qualitative approach (see Chapter 3)
    a. Identify the qualitative approach used—phenomenology, grounded theory, ethnography, exploratory-descriptive, or unspecified qualitative approach.
    b. Specific qualitative approach not identified:
        i. What aspects of the method, such as natural settings or coding, indicate that a qualitative approach was used (Creswell & Poth, 2018; Hall & Roussel, 2017; Munhall, 2012)?
        ii. Did the researcher provide a rationale for why a qualitative study was conducted (Creswell, 2014; Gray et al., 2017)?
    c. Did the researchers select a qualitative approach that produced data to meet the objectives or answer the research questions?

11. Sample (see Chapter 9)
    a. Is the sampling plan adequate to address the purpose of the study?
        i. If purposive sampling is used, does the researcher provide a rationale for the sample selection process?
        ii. If network or snowball sampling is used, does the researcher identify the networks used to obtain the sample and provide a rationale for their selection?
        iii. If theoretical sampling is used, does the researcher indicate how participants are selected to promote the generation of a theory?
    b. Are the sampling criteria identified and appropriate for the study?

12. If potential participants refused to participate, or participants did not complete the study, did the researcher acknowledge these issues as limitations?
13. Does the researcher discuss the quality of the data provided by the study participants?
14. Were the participants articulate, well informed, and willing to share information relevant to the study topic?
15. Did the sampling process produce saturation and verification of data in the area of the study?
16. Is the sample size adequate based on the scope of the study, nature of the topic, quality of the data, and study design?
17. How was informed consent obtained?
18. Was the process used for informed consent appropriate for the study population?
19. Setting
    a. What is the study setting?
    b. Is the setting appropriate for the study purpose?
    c. Did the setting in which data were collected protect the confidentiality and promote the comfort of the participants?

20. Data collection
    a. What data collection methods were used—interviews, focus groups, observation, or other sources?
    b. Interviews
        i. Were multiple interviews with the same person conducted, or were data collected once from each participant?
        ii. Were questions used during the interview or focus group relevant to the study's research objectives or questions (Gray et al., 2017; Maxwell, 2013)?
        iii. Did the interviews last long enough for the researcher to gather robust and thorough descriptions of the participants' perspectives?
    c. Focus group
        i. Was the size, composition, and length of the focus group adequate to promote group interaction and produce robust data?
        ii. Were questions used during the interview or focus group relevant to the study's research objectives or questions (Gray et al., 2017; Maxwell, 2013)?
    d. Observations
        i. Were observations conducted at times and for long enough periods to collect rich data that allowed for a thorough description of the culture, setting, or process of interest (Creswell & Poth, 2018; Wolf, 2012)?
        ii. Did the researcher make field notes or journal entries (Creswell, 2014; Miles, Huberman, & Saldaña, 2014)?
    e. How were data recorded during data collection?
    f. Was IRB approval obtained before data collection?

g. Did the researcher identify that participants might become upset during the collection of data? If so, what measures were in place to address the safety and emotional needs of the participants (Cowles, 1988; Maxwell, 2013)?

h. Were the data collection methods ethical?

21. Data analysis
    a. How were the data prepared for analysis?
    b. How were the data analyzed? Did the researcher cite a specific method of analysis and provide a primary source?
    c. Was computer-assisted qualitative data management software used during the analysis?
    d. Were the data analysis processes described thoroughly enough to be able to evaluate the logic of the researcher's decisions and support the rigor of the study?
    e. Which methods were used to increase the trustworthiness of the findings (e.g., verification of the accuracy of transcripts, immersion in the data, documentation of an audit trail [also known as the record of decisions that were made during data collection and analysis], member checking, and independent analysis of a portion of the data by another researcher) (Cohen & Crabtree, 2008; Hall & Roussel, 2017; Miles et al., 2014; Murphy & Yielder, 2010)?
    f. Were the measures to increase the trustworthiness of the study adequate to give the reader confidence in the findings (Cohen & Crabtree, 2008; Mackey, 2012; Wolf, 2012)?

Step 3: Evaluating the Credibility and Meaning of Study Findings

22. Interpretation of findings
    a. Describe the researcher's interpretation of findings.
    b. Were the findings linked to quotes or specific observations?
    c. Did the researcher address variations in the findings by relevant sample characteristics?
    d. Are the findings related back to the study framework (if applicable)?
    e. Are the findings consistent with previous research findings (Fawcett & Garity, 2009)?
    f. If the findings were unexpected, what explanations were given for why this may have occurred?

23. Limitations
    a. What study limitations did the researcher identify?
    b. Were there study limitations that the researcher did not acknowledge?
    c. Were the study limitations the result of factors under the researcher's control that could have been prevented, or were the limitations external factors over which the researcher had no control (Powers, 2015)?

24. Conclusions
    a. What conclusions did the researchers identify based on their interpretation of the study findings?
    b. Did the conclusions logically flow out of the findings?
    c. Did the researchers identify other settings or populations to whom the findings might be transferable or applied?

25. Nursing implications
    a. What implications for nursing practice were identified?
    b. Does the study expand nurses' understanding of the phenomenon studied? If so, how could the findings be used in nursing practice, theory, and education?
    c. How does this study support future knowledge development?

26. Future research
    a. What suggestions were identified for further study?
    b. Did the recommendations for further studies flow out of the findings?

27. Critical appraisal summary
    a. Review the components of the critique you just conducted. Consider the following to formulate your critical appraisal summary.
        i. Were all relevant components covered with adequate detail and clarity?
        ii. What were the study's greatest strengths and greatest weaknesses?

iii.   Were the rights of study participants protected (Creswell, 2014; Gray et al., 2017)?

iv.   Do you believe the study findings are valid? How much confidence can be placed in the study findings (Powers, 2015; Roller & Lavrakas, 2015)?

v.   The evaluation of a research report should also include a final discussion of the quality of the report. This discussion should include an expert opinion of the study's quality and contribution to nursing knowledge and practice (Melnyk & Fineout-Overholt, 2015; Melnyk et al., 2017; Powers, 2015).

References

Aberson, C. L. (2010). *Applied power analysis for the behavioral sciences.* New York, NY: Routledge Taylor & Francis.

Alligood, M. R. (2014). *Nursing theory: Utilization & application* (8th ed.). Maryland Heights, MO: Mosby Elsevier.

American Psychological Association (APA) (2010). *Publication manual of the American Psychological Association* (6th ed.). Washington, DC: Author.

Bialocerkowski, A., Klupp, N., & Bragge, P. (2010). Research methodology series: How to read and critically appraise a reliability article. *International Journal of Therapy and Rehabilitation, 17*(3), 114–120.

Brown, S. J. (2018). *Evidence-based nursing: The research-practice connection* (4th ed.). Sudbury, MA: Jones & Bartlett.

Chinn, P. L., & Kramer, M. K. (2015). *Integrated theory and knowledge development in nursing* (9th ed.). St. Louis, MO: Elsevier Mosby.

Cohen, D. J., & Crabtree, B. F. (2008). Evaluative criteria for qualitative research in health care: Controversies and recommendations. *Annals of Family Medicine, 6*(4), 331–339.

Cowles, K. (1988). Issues in qualitative research on sensitive topics. *Western Journal of Nursing Research, 10*(2), 163–179.

Creswell, J. W. (2014). *Research design: Qualitative, quantitative and mixed methods approaches* (3rd ed.). Thousand Oaks, CA: Sage.

Creswell, J. W., & Poth, C. (2018). *Qualitative inquiry & research design* (4th ed.). Thousand Oaks, CA: Sage.

DeVon, H. A., Block, M. E., Moyle-Wright, P., Ernst, D. M., Hayden, S. J., et al.(2007). A psychometric toolbox for testing validity and reliability. *Journal of Nursing Scholarship, 39*(2), 155–164.

Eymard, A. S., & Altmiller, G. (2016). Teaching nursing students the importance of treatment fidelity in intervention research: Students as interventionists. *Journal of Nursing Education, 55*(5), 288–291.

Fawcett, J., & Garity, J. (2009). *Evaluating research for evidence-based nursing practice.* Philadelphia, PA: F.A. Davis.

Gray, J. R., Grove, S. K., & Sutherland, S. (2017). *The practice of nursing research: Appraisal, synthesis, and generation of evidence* (8th ed.). St. Louis, MO: Elsevier Saunders.

Grove, S. K., & Cipher, D. J. (2017). *Statistics for nursing research: A workbook for evidence-based practice* (2nd ed.). St. Louis, MO: Elsevier.

Hall, H. R., & Roussel, L. A. (2017). *Evidence-based practice: An integrative approach to research, administration and practice* (2nd ed.). Burlington, MA: Jones & Bartlett.

Hart, C. (2009). *Doing a literature review: Releasing the social science imagination.* Thousand Oaks, CA: Sage Publications.

Hoare, Z., & Hoe, J. (2013). Understanding quantitative research: Part 2. *Nursing Standard (Royal College of Nursing [Great Britain]), 27*(18), 48–55.

Mackey, M. (2012). Evaluation of qualitative research. In P. L. Munhall (Ed.), *Nursing research: A qualitative perspective* (pp. 517–531). (5th ed.). Sudbury, MA: Jones & Bartlett.

Maxwell, J. (2013). *Qualitative research design: An interactive approach* (3rd ed.). Thousand Oaks, CA: Sage.

Melnyk, B. M., & Fineout-Overholt, E. (Eds.). (2015). *Evidence-based practice in nursing & healthcare: A guide to best practice.* (3rd ed.). Philadelphia, PA: Wolters Kluwer.

Melnyk, B. M., Gallagher-Ford, E., & Fineout-Overholt, E. (2017). *Implementing evidence-based practice competencies in healthcare: A practical guide for improving quality, safety, & outcomes.* Indianapolis, IN: Sigma Theta Tau International.

Miles, M., Huberman, A., & Saldaña, J. (2014). *Qualitative data analysis: A methods sourcebook* (3rd ed.). Thousand Oaks, CA: Sage.

Munhall, P. L. (2012). *Nursing research: A qualitative perspective* (5th ed.). Sudbury, MA: Jones & Bartlett.

Murphy, F., & Yielder, J. (2010). Establishing rigor in qualitative radiography. *Radiography, 16*(1), 62–67.

O'Mathúna, D. P., & Fineout-Overholt, E. (2015). Critically appraising quantitative evidence for clinical decision making. In B. M. Melnyk, & E. Fineout-Overholt (Eds.), *Evidence-based practice in nursing & healthcare: A guide to best practice* (pp. 87–138). (2nd ed.). Philadelphia, PA: Lippincott Williams & Wilkins.

Plichta, S. B., & Kelvin, E. (2013). *Munro's statistical methods for health care research* (6th ed.). Philadelphia, PA: Lippincott Williams & Wilkins.

Powers, B. A. (2015). Critically appraising qualitative evidence for clinical decision making. In B. M. Melnyk, & E. Fineout-Overholt (Eds.), *Evidence-based practice in nursing & healthcare: A guide to best practice* (pp. 139–168). (2nd ed.). Philadelphia, PA: Lippincott Williams & Wilkins.

Roller, M., & Lavrakas, P. (2015). *Applied qualitative research design: A total quality framework approach.* New York, NY: Guilford Press.

Ryan-Wenger, N. A. (2017). Precision, accuracy, and uncertainty of biophysical measurements for clinical research and practice. In C. F. Waltz, O. L. Strickland, & E. R. Lenz (Eds.), *Measurement in nursing and health research* (pp. 371–383). (4th ed.). New York, NY: Springer.

Shadish, W. R., Cook, T. D., & Campbell, D. T. (2002). *Experimental and quasi-experimental designs for generalized causal inference.* Chicago, IL: Rand McNally.

Smith, M. J., & Liehr, P. R. (2014). *Middle range theory for nursing* (3rd ed.). New York, NY: Springer.

Waltz, C. F., Strickland, O. L., & Lenz, E. R. (2017). *Measurement in nursing and health research* (5th ed.). New York, NY: Springer.

Wolf, M. (2012). Ethnography: The method. In P. L. Munhall (Ed.), *Nursing research: A qualitative perspective* (pp. 285–338). (5th ed.). Sudbury, MA. Jones & Bartlett.